The History
of Chinese Dance

TRADITIONAL CHINESE ARTS AND CULTURE

The History of Chinese Dance

Wang Kefen

FOREIGN LANGUAGES PRESS   BEIJING

First edition 1985

Translated into English by Ke Ruibo

ISBN 0-8351-1186-5

Published by the Foreign Languages Press
24 Baiwanzhuang Road, Beijing, China
Printed by the Foreign Languages Printing House
19 West Chegongzhuang Road, Beijing, China
Distributed by China International Book Trading Corporation
(Guoji Shudian) P.O. Box 399, Beijing, China

Printed in the People's Republic of China

Contents

Chapter One
An Investigation into Primitive Dance — 1

Chapter Two
Music and Dance in Slave Society — 7

Chapter Three
The Rise of Folk Song and Dance and Dancing Girls — 15

Chapter Four
Han Dynasty "Variety Shows" and Dances — 20

Chapter Five
The Exchange of Song and Dance Between Different Nationalities — 39

Chapter Six
The Tang Dynasty—Golden Age for Dance in Ancient Times — 48

Chapter Seven
Song Folk Dance and "Dance Troupes" — 66

Chapter Eight
Dance and Traditional Opera During the Ming and Qing Dynasties — 77

Chapter Nine
Dances of the National Minorities — 89

Appendix
Thirty Years of Continuation and Development — 100

CHAPTER ONE

An Investigation into Primitive Dance

Dance is the art of portraying a certain state of mind through the ordered rhythmic actions and configurations of the human body. The *Book of Rites*, a Confucian classic describing ceremonial in ancient China, mentions in the "Notes on Music" that sound issues from Man's innermost being and that Man's feelings are excited by the external world. When his heart is thus stirred, "voice" issues forth; through the interaction of these "voices", a changed and regulated "sound" appears which is then called "tone" (music); when it is performed and danced to with shields, axes, bird-feathers, flags (decorated with yak tails long ago), the result is "music". What was then referred to as music thus included song and dance as well. According to the *Book of Odes*, the earliest compilation of songs and poems in China, "If words do not suffice, then sigh; if sighing fails, then sing; if singing is not enough, then let your arms and legs dance it." Clearly then, even 2,000 years ago poetry, song and dance were considered as arts for expressing Man's ideas and feelings.

Dance Depicting Physical Work

There were no classes in Primitive Society and thus no exploitation. Men lived in groups and went hunting together. Happy at their catch of birds and animals which would provide food and clothing, they would gather together on their return from the hunt and dance to the beat of a stone implement like a chime in a rhythmic imitation of the birds' and animals' movements and form. The so called "Birds and Animals Hop in Step", "The Phoenix Comes to Pay Homage", "To the Beat of a Stone, All the Animals Dance" recorded in the *Book of History*, a compilation of records from ancient Chinese history, is just such a lively reflection of hunting life.

"All the Animals Dance" was not merely a re-enactment in celebration of victory or the hunting life. It is also a reflection of the fact that the elders passed on knowledge for survival to the young people by teaching them how to differentiate various birds and animals as well as how to catch them. Passed down and elaborated on by countless generations, the nationalities living in China now have a rich and lively repertoire of dances depicting every kind of animal.

A Neolithic earthenware bowl with dance designs (see fig. 1) was unearthed in the village grave at Shangsunjiazhai, Datong County, Qinghai Province. On its inner lip there are four parallel bands. Above them are drawn the figures of three groups of dancers. Each group consists of five people, their heads and bodies slightly inclined. The extended arms of the couple on the edge of the groups are drawn as two lines, possibly to depict a waving motion. They are danc-

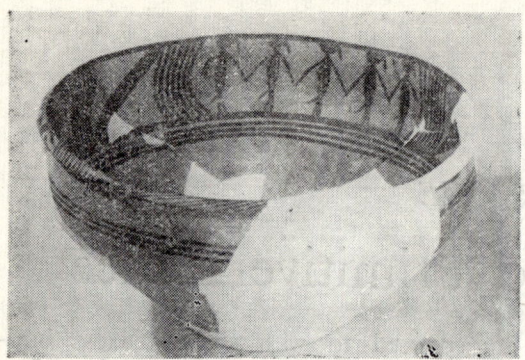
1. Neolithic earthenware bowl with dance designs. Unearthed at Datong County, Qinghai.

ing together hand in hand in an orderly fashion. Accounts in poetry and essays from the Han (206 B.C.-A.D. 220) and Tang (A.D. 618-907) dynasties onwards indicate that people would sing and tramp their feet to the rhythm as they linked arms in an uninhibited dance which had no fixed number of participants. It was a traditional form of recreational group dance enjoyed by the Han and many other nationalities. The discovery of the earthenware bowl with dance designs proves that far back during the period of Primitive Society the forebears of the Chinese people had already created this kind of group dance form. Braids or ornaments hang down at an angle from the heads of the dancers on the bowl, they all have a small tail behind them — doubtless decorations for enacting various animals! The image of early man acting out "All the Animals Dance" is portrayed in a lively way and since it is the oldest such depiction of dancing so far discovered is of great value.

On the upper half of a Warring States pot with handles in the form of animal heads, each holding a ring in its mouth, are carvings of a hunting scene (see fig. 2). On the lower half are engraved figures enacting a dance in bird form. They are all in a line, facing the same way and wearing long plumes as headdresses, their arms look like birds' wings. Tail decorations stick out behind. It is in the tradition of primitive animal dance and has points of similarity with the figures on the bowl with dance designs.

From the distant past down to the present day the various nationalities in China have had many dances imitating the behaviour of birds and animals such as the lion dance, dragon dance, peacock dance, halcyon dance, mynah dance, thrush dance and others. Traditional dance terminology also has a large number of movements named after bird and animal actions. Examples are "Pair of Flying Swallows", "The Giant Roc Spreads Its Wings", "Tiger Jumping", "Pouncing Tiger", "Black Dragon Shakes the Columns", and "Step of the Scorpion".

Too numerous to mention, these terms in both ordinary and figurative dance are closely connected with working life such as hunting.

As animal husbandry and agriculture gradually developed, the scope of Man's life broadened and consequently the songs and dances which reflected that life became richer. Ancient Chinese legend tells of a kind of song and dance called "The Music of Getian" which had a set structure and form. Three people carrying oxtails tramped to the rhythm of the music singing and dancing. It was divided into eight sections: possibly in the first section our primitive forebears sang the praises of Man himself; the second section was in praise of their totem symbol, the crane; the third was a supplication for the plants to grow well; the fourth prayed for a good harvest; homage was paid to Heaven in the fifth; the next section praised God's munificence in aiding Man; the seventh thanked the Earth for her bounty; and the eighth and final section looked forward to a proliferation of animals so Man would be provided with food and clothing in abundance. Song and dance were integrated with working life and also reflected the undeveloped religious consciousness of our forebears — that is to say veneration of Heaven, Earth and Ancestors.

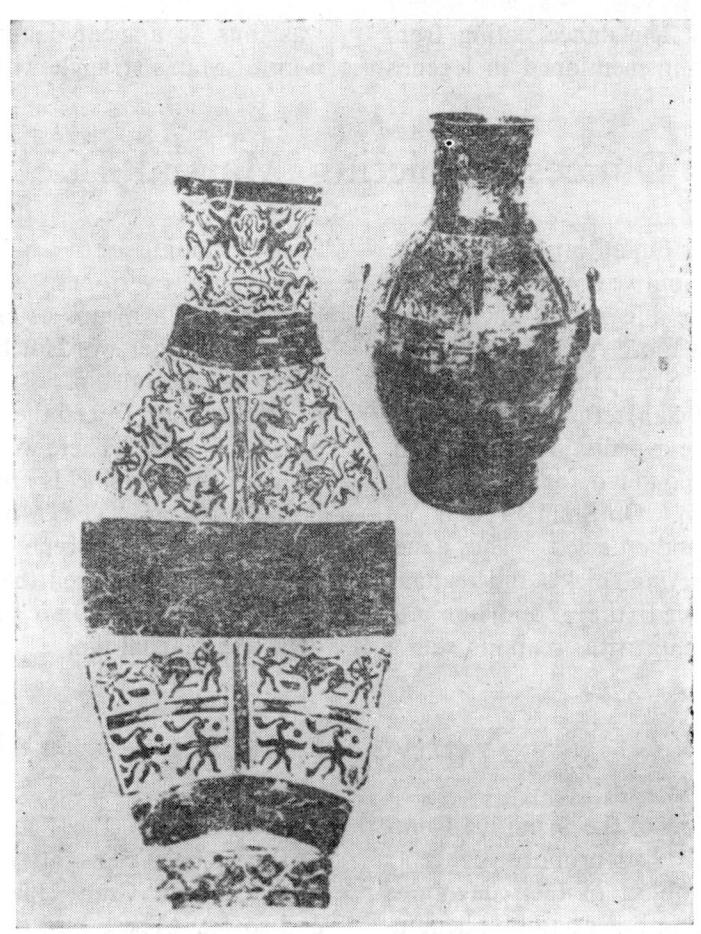

2. Warring States pot with animal heads, each holding a ring in its mouth, and hunting motifs. The original and a copy of the design.

Ancient Dances for Keeping Fit

The *Lü's Spring and Autumn Annals*, a work typical of the Eclectic school, was jointly compiled at the end of the Warring States Period (475-221 B.C.) by court scholars brought together by a Qin minister called Lü Buwei. One chapter in it "On Ancient Music" tells of a legend that there was a great flood in ancient times under Yinkang. "The waterways were blocked, the river did not follow its course." The people suffered from the damp and cold so "their physique became number and stiff". A dance was created for them to do so they could develop their bodies and thus recover. It served as an exercise. In fact, traditional Chinese dance is closely connected with the martial arts which trains fighting skills as well as being for fitness. Some dances have developed directly from the martial arts which themselves of course include much beautiful choreography. Others like the "Sabre Dance" can be traced from actual sword fighting right down to its form as an embellished artistic dance. There are many similar examples. The dance dating from the time of Yinkang mentioned in legends was thus an ancient dance for keeping fit, born of Man's struggle with Nature.

Dances Depicting Martial Life

War would break out at times between the various clans in Primitive Society. The fact there was a battle life meant there were dances reflecting it too. A legend says that during the time of Shun, the Youmiao (the name of an ancient clan) refused to surrender, so Yu led a punitive expedition against them. They fought the Youmiao for 30 days but failed to beat them. On Shun's orders Yu withdrew his men and returned. They danced for 70 days carrying shields and feathers which finally scared the Youmiao into submission. Dancing with weapons was a form of training for the soldiers which carried threatening overtones. But dancing with feathers was a means of expressing "refinement", in other words it bore a message of peace and friendship. By taking these two measures, Shun forced the Youmiao to come over to his side. There were other legendary dances in which shields and battleaxes were borne such as "The Music of Xingtian" or the "Wrestling Scene" which originated from the fight between the Yellow Emperor and Chi You. They are all ancient dances depicting martial life.

Votive Dances

During the period of the Primitive Commune, Man already had primitive concepts of religion. The object of their devotions was often an animal or other natural phenomenon. They were presumed to be their own ancestors and were made clan totems. An example occurs in the first general biographical history in China the *Records of the Historian* compiled by Sima Qian in the 1st century B.C. during the Western Han. The Yellow Emperor fought both Chi You and the Emperor Yan at different times. He trained bears, tigers and other mythical animals — in fact clans named after wild animals, to take part in the fight. A further example occurs in *Zuoqiu Ming's Chronicles*, a compilation dating from the early years of the Warring States which relates the history of the Spring and Autumn Period (770-476 B.C.). The general meaning of the passage is that during the Spring and Autumn Period a man called Tan Zi claimed he was descended from the Shaohao tribe which "named their clans after birds" so there were Phoenix, Crane, Black Bird, Red Bird and so on. These bird names all stood for a clan. Moreover, judging by some legends, every clan had its own representative songs and dances used in praise of their own clan's heroes or as homage to Heaven and Earth and the Ancestors.

Yet another story goes that Yao, the leader of the tribal alliance in primitive times, ordered Zhi to compose music. Zhi mimicked the sounds of mountain, stream and forest in his work. The rhythm was beaten out on pottery drums and stone shards (later chime stones). An extra 10 strings were added to the five-string lute. When it was sung in performance "all the animals" began to dance. It was known as the "Dazhang" and was used by Yao to pay homage to God. The *History of Lu*, a description of historical events during legendary times in China compiled by Luo Bi in the Southern Song (1127-1279) adds that the eight-string lute was increased to twenty-three strings during the reign of Yao, and that the "Xianchi dance was composed" "for the pleasure of God". By contrast, the *Rites of the Zhou Dynasty*, first written down during the Warring States Period, maintains that the 'Xianchi' dates from the time of the Yellow Emperor but was enlarged and revised under Yao.

The legends described above indicate that the "Dazhang" dance was probably composed during the reign of Yao though it drew on the "Xianchi" which went back to the time of the Yellow Emperor. Originally, the "Xianchi" was a constellation in the western sky believed by people then to have influence over the crops. The dance was probably performed in homage to it as a prayer for good harvests.

Tradition holds that the "Shao" was a dance dating from the time of Yao's successor Shun. There was a terrible flood then so Shun ordered Yu to carry out flood prevention work on the rivers. Yu took charge of dredging the rivers, and building irrigation canals to improve agriculture. The work took 13 years and though he passed by his home on three occasions during that time he did not go in. The *Records of the Historian* says that a vast celebration was held in honour of Yu's success in flood control and Shun's benevolent rule. Shun handed over power to Yu and Kui composed the music, each clan performing their own dances. Then the "birds and beasts" bounded forth and by the time the "Shao" had reached the ninth section, the "phoenix" started to dance along with "all the animals". According to the findings of historians, Kui was probably the musically gifted chieftain of the Youreng clan who later became Shun's court musician. It thus seems likely that the "Shao" was his work or a compilation he made incorporating traditional songs and dances of the Youreng.

The "Shao" was a famous ancient dance. According to *Zuoqiu Ming's Chronicles* Prince Jizha from the Kingdom of Wu saw a performance of an early Zhou (11th century B.C.) arrangement of the "Shao" at Lu in 544 B.C. during the Spring and Autumn Period. He was quite moved and praised it as a "truly wonderful piece of music that transcends all". The *Analects* (a record of Confucius' words and deeds written by his disciples and later followers) also mentions it. In 517 B.C., it says, Confucius heard the "Shao" in the Kingdom of Qi and for three months he did not know the taste of meat. He remarked that he had not realized the "Shao" could so affect people. Confucius also praised it as a consummate work. Though legends from the Spring and Autumn Period cannot be completely trusted, after all they come some 1,000 years after the Neolithic Period when it is said to have been written, the Shao was nevertheless much enjoyed by people of the time. Through being handed down over many years, the Shao continued to gain in richness to end up as the rounded and beautiful dance it was for the period.

Legend says the "Daxia" was a dance in praise of Yu of the Xia. Yu's exploits have already been described. When the water courses had finally been dredged and the floods brought under control, the people living then ordered Gao Tao to compose the Daxia in celebration of Yu's great achievement in taming them. In Zhou times (11th century-256 B.C.) 64 people would take part. They danced bare-chested wearing fur caps and plain white skirts — the dress of manual workers. A man called Ji Zha from the Kingdom of Wu saw a performance of the early Zhou arrangement of the Daxia at the Kingdom of Lu in 544 B.C. He praised it as being "Beautiful! A depiction of work not virtues." It is possible that movements imitating flood control were used in the dance. Early Man's courage in overcoming the trials of Nature is expressed through its fairly simple dance idiom.

For the most part there are no reliable records of dance in Primitive Society that can be consulted. We can only pick out those key elements from ancient legends that are logical and fit in with the rules of social development and subject them to analytical research. The primitive dances in such legends are all closely connected with Man's life — whether it be work, battle or worship — and are a direct reflection of it.

CHAPTER TWO

Music and Dance in Slave Society

After a long period of development, Primitive Society gradually evolved into Slave Society.

Until the time of Yu of the Xia, clan chieftains had been chosen by election. With Yu's transfer of power to his son Qi, there began the dynastic system of Chinese history. The Xia Dynasty after Qi took control had already entered into Slave Society. This period in China lasted through the Shang (about the 16th-11th century B.C.), Western Zhou (11th century-770 B.C.) and Spring and Autumn Period — more than 1,600 years.

Shaman Dances and Dances of Exorcism

Man had no means of understanding many natural phenomena in ancient times. Such things were thought to be cloaked in mystery, spirits governed everything. So when there were any disasters or problems, the gods were consulted and invoked for protection. The first people to perform such sacrificial and divinatory offices were called "shamans". It was superstitiously believed that the shamans could communicate with the gods by becoming their incarnation and acting as a mouthpiece. When practising their sorcery, shamans tried to propitiate the gods by singing and dancing which we shall call shaman dances.

The earliest Chinese writing, carved on turtle shells or animal bones, is known as "oracle bone inscriptions". On such inscriptions the character for dance (now 舞) was written as 兩 — in the shape of a dancer holding oxtails (see fig.3). As mentioned earlier, that was one form of primitive dance. The words "Duolao dance" appear in oracle bone inscriptions. Historical research indicates that Duolao was probably the name of a shaman. The people of the Shang were consulting the gods by divination to see

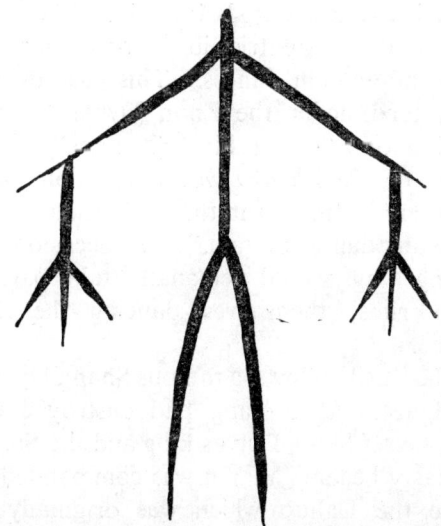

3. Copy of the Shang oracle bone inscription for the word "dance".

whether it was propitious to ask the shaman Duolao to dance for rain.

To increase their control over the slaves, the slave-owning class strengthened the slave system regime. By use of the supernatural to keep the population down they were making conscious efforts to heighten the religious awareness of the people. As a result, shamanistic practices were very widespread. The Shang kings claimed to be descendants of the gods so the spirits had to be consulted on any matter, however trifling — though of course when it really came to choosing a course of action, it was they themselves who decided. This was simply a means by which the slave-owning aristocracy abused the name of the gods to control and subdue the people. As the shamans were supposed to be able to commune with the gods their status was fairly high and they held considerable power. For example during the Shang Dynasty there were some who became acting Ministers of State.

Agriculture was the most important sector of the Shang economy, consequently success or failure of the crops had considerable repercussions. Whenever there was a prolonged drought, the people of the Shang would invoke the gods for rain. There are as a result many entries in the oracle inscriptions about rain dances. This custom was continued under the Zhou Dynasty. The section on "Controlling Shamans" in the *Rites of the Zhou Dynasty* mentions that "If there is drought in the land, then all the shamans dance for rain." On occasion the Shang kings would personally take part in such rites, themselves dancing the rain dance.

The "Dahuo" was a famous Shang Dynasty dance. After Tang had destroyed the Xia, he set himself up as king and the Shang Dynasty began. Yi Yin was commanded to write the Dahuo which was originally to celebrate the founding of the dynasty. On Tang's death his descendants adopted it as a dance of homage to their ancestors. There are records of this in the oracle bone inscriptions where Tang's descendants used divination to see whether the "Dahuo" should be employed in such rites.

Shang government was theocratic, the shaman dances were to propitiate the gods. However as society developed these dances gradually became for people's enjoyment as well. The *Book of History* says that they were "often danced in the palaces, sung drunkenly in the halls and were known as sorcery" then and put them on a par with promiscuity and unrest as one of the three trends that had to be stopped. But why did people want to dance all the time and why were they so keen on singing? Just for pleasure. Shaman dances for entertainment slowly developed in later generations and as time went on people believed less and less the rubbish that shamans could commune with the gods. During the Warring States Period, Ximen Bao, a statesman from the Kingdom of Wei, was sent to Ye as county magistrate. Sometimes the River Zhangshui would overflow and flood. There was an old custom in the area whereby the shaman chose a beautiful maiden and flung her into the river every year saying that the floods could be alleviated by giving a wife to the God of the River. She used the opportunity to extort money from the people. Ximen Bao threw the shaman and her disciples into the river thus destroying the myth. He then mobilized the people to cut 12 water courses in order to change the Zhangshui River from being a threat into a benefit through irrigation. The area's agriculture improved accordingly. The tale of Ximen Bao alleviating local suffering has been handed down for generations.

Under the Jin (A.D. 265-420) two female shamans, Chen Zhu and Zhang Dan, used to dress in gorgeous clothes and were expert singers and dancers. Their shaman dance consisted of light, graceful steps with circling and turning motions. By co-ordinating their movements they could heighten the emotional interplay. Some acrobatic-like pieces were also included. Yet apart from the mysterious ambience of the performance, it in no way differed from those given by dancing girls of the time.

Shaman ritual also preserved dances which have become folk traditions such as the Single Drum from the Northeast (also known as the Taiping Drum). Though originally one of the shaman dances it gradually evolved over the years into a folk dance for festivals. After Liberation in 1949, dancers re-arranged it. By cutting out its superstitious religious overtones and highlighting its positive aspects they turned it into a popular dance number.

Exorcism was a ceremony used in ancient times for driving out evil spirits and epidemics. We shall call the dances performed on such occasions "Dances of Exorcism". The dancers would wear masks and dance frenziedly to drive clear away all malevolent "Demons of Pestilence" or "Devils". Its origins date a long way back, there are even records from the Zhou Dynasty. It enjoyed an unbroken tradition of several thousand years. On every New Year's Eve and at other seasons, the custom of performing dances of exorcism was observed not just by the Court but among the populace too. The "Picture of a Great Exorcism" dating from the Song (960-1279) (see fig.4) depicts 12 figures wearing various kinds of masks. They carry everyday household implements such as brooms, fans, ladles and winnowing pans as dance props. The cheerful and lively scene shows them in a twisting snake formation which advances as they call and shout along the line. It is valuable material for the study of ancient folk "Dances of Exorcism".

After Liberation, dancers visited Guangxi and Jiangxi to collect ancient folk dances. The Dances of Exorcism were in a simple unsophisticated style with strong, crude movements. The spirit of the people in having the courage to overcome evil in the pursuit of a happy life is embodied in their lusty humour.

Dancing Slaves

The dancing slaves were song and dance artistes who performed solely for the entertainment of the slave masters. Dance had developed from being a spontaneous group activity for personal enjoyment into an entertainment performed for other people — marking the gradual entry of dance into the realms of a performing art. Dancing slaves were the main force behind this.

On coming to power the first ruler of the slave era, Qi of the Xia, is said to have quite openly appropriated the Shao — then highly revered as a dance of homage to the ancestors — for his own amusement. He even created the myth that he personally brought the Shao down from Heaven to be performed amongst Mankind. The *Mohist Canon* reprimands him for "taking all kinds of arranged dance forms" for his own entertainment though there have been different interpretations as to the exact meaning of these lines.

Another legend says that a ruler at the end of the Xia Dynasty — Jie — kept 30,000 dancing girls (though this may be an exaggeration) and that the performances were so loud they could be heard from afar. He thought dances should be "the bigger the better, the more the merrier". In other words he went in for extravagance and ostentation.

The story is also told that Zhou, the last ruler of the Shang, made the lives of the slaves working for him even harder in his pursuit of

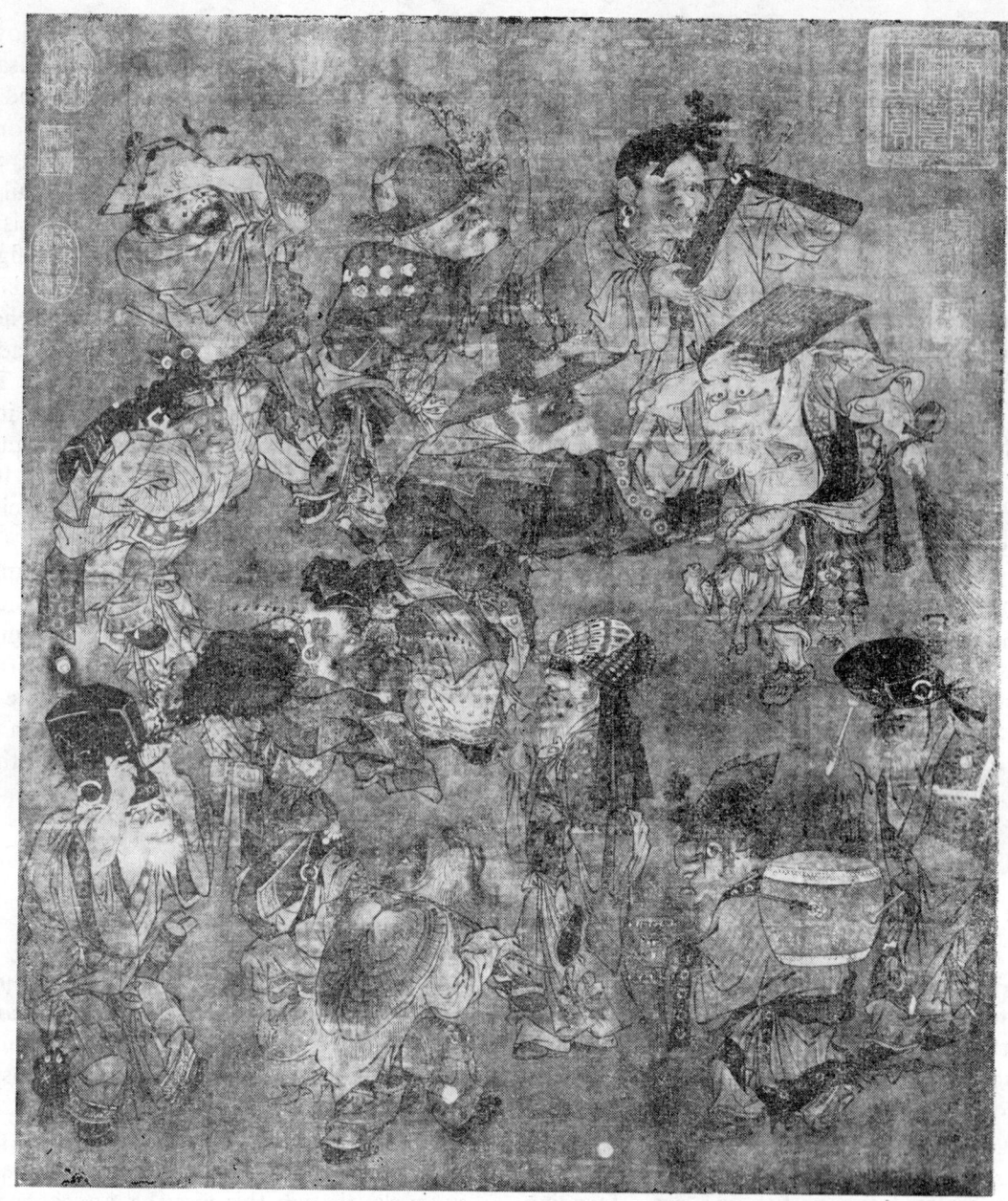
4. Song picture of a "Great Exorcism".

pleasure. He was a profligate spendthrift. "Vast dancing shows were held on the sand dunes" so it can be gathered that the dances already had unsavoury overtones. However it is possible that there were consequent improvements and innovations in performing technique due to the ruling classes' increased demands on dance as a form of entertainment.

While still alive the slave masters made the slaves' lot a very hard one, enjoying complete control over any material or spiritual wealth they created as well as their very lives. Even after the slave-owners died, large numbers of slaves were killed to be buried with the dead in the mistaken belief that they would continue to serve their masters in the next world. In 1950 the large tomb of a slave-owning noble from the Shang Dynasty was unearthed at Wuguan Village in Anyang, Henan Province. The corpses of twenty-four women were found on the west side of the coffin chamber. Funerary objects included a large chime stone beautifully decorated with a relief of a snarling tiger. The sound of the chime was still strong and clear, a masterpiece by artisans of the time. Also unearthed were three small copper dagger-axes. The fact there were vestiges of silk and bird feathers shows that some of the women buried with the deceased were dancing girls.

The dancing slaves were just like the slaves who made the exquisite bronze ware. Although they composed beautiful songs and dances for their masters' enjoyment they could be slaughtered at any time, lacking even any rights over their own existence.

The Setting Up of the System of Court Dance

Zhou was originally a vassal state under the Shang but it gradually became stronger as time went on. After much preparation the Zhou took advantage of a period of acute contradictions within the Shang Court to ally themselves wity tribes from neighbouring states and launch an attack. Their morale was high on the march, they sang and danced. During a battle at Muye the slaves in the Shang army rose up before the ranks and in co-ordination with the Zhou turned their spears on their masters to wipe out the Shang for ever. In about the 11th century B.C. a powerful slave state was established — the Western Zhou.

On assuming power, besides adopting a string of political and military measures, the Zhou paid particular attention to thought control. They did all they could to publicize the fact that they had received the Mandate of Heaven to crush the Shang and punish its king Zhou, that they were destined to rule the people.

To consolidate their rule, they strengthened the concept of rank as much as possible and worked out a system of ritual music and dance. During the early years of the dynasty songs and dances typical of various clans under previous dynasties are said to have been collated and edited under the direction of Dan, the Duke of Zhou. They were used in important ceremonies like paying homage to Heaven, Earth and Ancestors and at court celebrations.

The palace set up a fairly large body for song and dance which came under the Director of Music, who supervised all such matters, taught the noble children the rudiments of song and dance and instructed them in the dances for various rituals.

Both the "Six Dances" and the "Small Dances" which were famous in ancient times are supposed to have been established during the early Zhou as dances for votive rituals. The "Six Dances" were as follows: first came the "Yunmen" said to date back to the time of the Yellow Emperor and used by the Zhou for paying homage to the Sky God; secondly the "Xianchi" which legend holds came from the same period too but had been revised by Yao, and was performed under the Zhou for sacrifice to the Earth God; next was the "Shao", a dance fabled to go back to the time of Shun but later used in homage to the Gods of the Four Directions (or some say the sun, moon, stars and sea); fourthly the

"Daxia" believed to date back to Yu of the Xia which served in devotions to the mountains and rivers; fifthly the "Dahuo", a dance said to have originated in the Emperor Tang's reign during the Xia Dynasty, but was adopted in Zhou times for veneration of female ancestors; finally came the "Dawu" which was in praise of King Wu of the Zhou, it was used in ancestor worship. The first five dances all carried on from previous dynasties so here we will concentrate on discussing the Dawu.

The Dawu was a tribute to the military exploits of King Wu of the Zhou in his expedition against King Zhou. The battle then gained the support of the slaves so had a certain progressive significance. This could also be the main reason for the dance's high standing in history.

The Dawu was a product of the early years of the Western Zhou when the country was being built up. Confucius saw a performance some 500 years later after it had gone through many changes prompting him to discuss the general state of the performance with Bin Moujia. Extracts from the Dawu are also mentioned in some ancient works. From these extracts we can see that the dance was divided into six parts. To begin with there was a long section of drumming, probably as a prelude to the dance. The dancers assembled ready to go on stage. Next, after trouping out from the north side armed with shields and other weapons, they stood in a well-arranged group singing in long drawn out voices. In the second part it switched to a vigorous dance showing the scene at the battlefront. On either side of the troupe, people rang battle bells (for proclaiming war) at which the group split into two rows. Making fierce stabbing movements, they came forward dancing to represent the annihilation of the Shang. After the destruction of the Shang they advanced again towards the south. The fourth section showed how the border territories in the south had already been pacified. The troupe then split into two lines once more to symbolize the assistance provided by the Duke of Zhou on the left and the Duke of Zhao on the right to the rule of the Zhou king. They went on to give a slick performance of all kinds of complicated group formations. The rhythm quickened and they reformed as an orderly troupe. Next the dancers squatted in a meditative pose to depict the country's attainment of good government. They finally regrouped to demonstrate their respect to the sovereign and with that the dance came to a close. Though handed down over a long period of time it does seem that the Dawu preserved a certain martial air. Dances with weapons had already appeared in the primitive dances of legend so the "Dawu" must have been a larger-scale, improved version of these but with a more cohesive and complicated structure.

The "Small Dances" consisted of six forms of sacrificial dance to be performed by young aristocrats in the Western Zhou. First came the "Dance with Coloured Silk". The dancers held full plumes or coloured silk as they paid obeisance to the Earth and Grain Gods (ancient symbols of state power). Secondly, the "Feather Dance" — participants carried bent feathers (possibly half-splayed plumes) in a dance similar to the Feather Dance of the Dian nationality. Performances were in tribute to ancestral temples or the Gods of the Four Quarters. Thirdly, the "Imperial Dance", for which the dancers wore feather hats and green feather costumes or held coloured plumes. It was performed in homage to the Gods of the Four Quarters or as a rain dance. Fourthly, the "Banner Dance" where the dancers carried yak tails in sacrificial rites at the Biyong — a Zhou seat of learning. Fifthly, the "Shield Dance", the dancers carried shields, was danced for military purposes or in obeisance to the Hills and Rivers. Sixthly, the "Dance of the People" which used no props and was danced empty-handed with sleeve actions. It was performed in honour of the stars or ancestral temples.

Dances where animal tails or plumage were carried related to hunting life, a tradition from previous generations. Many objects uncovered at Shizhaishan at Jinning in Yunnan reflect conditions under Western Han slave society near Lake Dianchi. They prove that certain of the ritual systems of the western Zhou slave society were the same as those of the slave society in the Lake Dianchi area. The decorations on the copper implements unearthed there serve as an example. These are lively depictions of dance scenes in which feather hats were worn and plumage and shields carried (see figs. 5, 6 and 7). They are valuable reference materials for the study of ancient dance.

In addition, there were the music and dances of national minorities at the Zhou court such as the "Music of the Border Tribes" and "Free Form Music" of folk

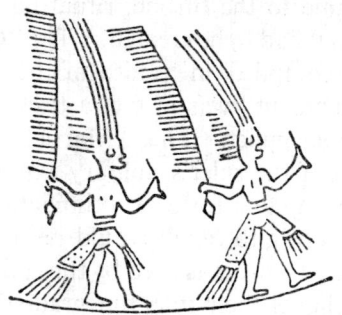

6. Dian feather dance from the Western Han. Copy of a detail.

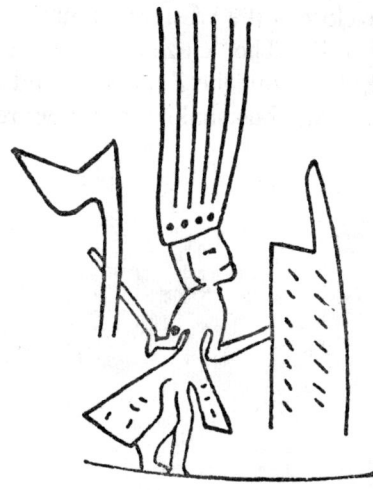

7. Dancer with shield and battleaxe. Copy of a detail on a bronze drum from Jinning, Yunnan.

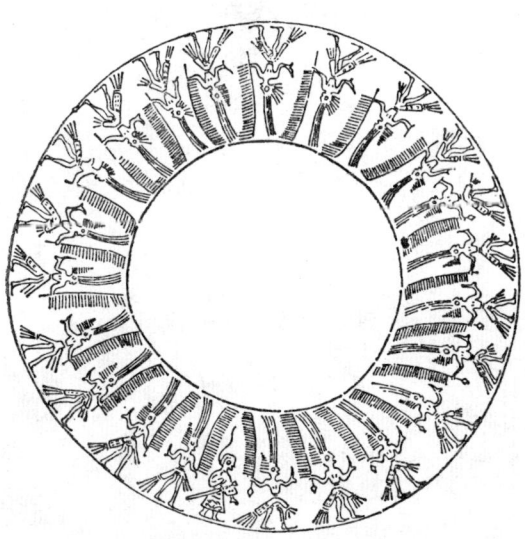

5. Dian feather dance of the Western Han. A copy of decorations on the lid of a bronze utensil for storing cowrie shells.

origin. They were mostly performed at banquets. Ranking was strictly laid down under the Zhou and each grade had its own specific dance. For example, the royal dance troupe consisted of 64 people in eight rows of eight, those of feudal lords 36 in six rows of six and high ranking officials 16, four rows of four.

Down through the ages succeeding generations of feudal rulers praised the Zhou system of court ritual as being "Music of the Early Kings" and "sublime music". Whenever there was a change of dynasty or a new emperor came to the throne, ritual dance and ceremonial had to be created. The "Civilian Dance" compiled in praise of the ruler's "enlightenment" was in fact a trick to keep the people quiet. The "Martial Dance" in praise of the ruler's military exploits was little more than a form of intimidation since anyone daring to revolt would be put down by force. Dance was used by the ruling class to consolidate their rule, but gradually such music and dances became a hackneyed and uninteresting ritual over the long period of feudal society. Even the ruling classes did not enjoy them.

At the close of the Western Zhou there was a slave revolt. The "citizens of the country" rebelled, drove out the Zhou king and killed the aristocrats thus shaking the cruel regime of the slave system to its very foundations. The Western Zhou came to an end with the assassination of King You of the Zhou at the foot of Mount Lishan. In 770 B.C. King Ping moved the capital eastwards from Hao (present-day Xi'an, Shaanxi) to Luoyi (now Luoyang in Henan). which became known in history as the Eastern Zhou (770-256 B.C.). However from then on the Zhou Dynasty lost its power or control over the feudal lords and Chinese history entered a period of great change and turmoil — the Spring and Autumn and Warring States periods. The ritual system of court dance and music established to shore up the rule of the slave system collapsed along with it, but folk song and dance, fresh and lively, flourished.

CHAPTER THREE

The Rise of Folk Song and Dance and Dancing Girls

Due to the gradual formation of feudal productive relations between the Spring and Autumn and Warring States periods, the forces of production were liberated. Agriculture, handicrafts and commerce grew. Along with this economic development, culture and art flourished as never before. The hackneyed dances associated with the "Music of the Early Kings" during the Western Zhou fell into disfavour whereas folk song and dance known as "Plain Dance" or "Dances of Zheng and Wei" gradually grew in popularity.

The "White Elm by the East Gate" in the "Airs of Chen" from the *Book of Odes* gives vivid descriptions of the vogue for folk song and dance in the Kingdom of Chen (the area of modern Henan and Anhui).

> There is a white elm by the East Gate,
> And on the hillock an oak,
> The maidens from Zizhong's house
> Come beneath the trees to dance.
>
> The time chosen is right,
> On the southern plain,
> No need to spin flax,
> Come to market and dance.
>
> Good times go quickly,
> Find pleasure where you can,
> You're like a flower on a thornbush,
> Giving me nothing but prickles.

At festivals, the young danced happily together singing of their true love — a custom which continues to this day in many of the national minority areas of China.

Another song, the "Wanqiu", also contains verses describing folk dances from the Kingdom of Chen. It says that people living at the foot of Wanqiu Mountain danced their hearts out to the beat of the drum come rain or shine. They either carried feathers or wore them on their heads.

Sorcery was rife in the state of Chu (the area of present-day Hunan). The great poet Qu Yuan crafted his "Nine Odes" from folk songs and dances used in votive rites there. The "Nine Odes" gives us an idea of some of the features of popular shaman song and dance then.

It was divided into 11 sections altogether. The "Great Emperor of the East" describes the scene at the start of the obeisances. On an auspicious day people flocked to pay homage to the god (the Great Emperor of the East). Dressed in heavily ornamented ceremonial robes, the shamans would troop out carrying long swords to drive away evil spirits. The altar was filled with sacrificial objects and the long drawn out votive singing began. Sorceresses, beautifully made up, danced and sang a lilting accompaniment to the intricate music. They then proceeded to pay obeisance to the Lady of the Clouds, the "Goddess of the Xiangshui River" and "Lady of the Xiangshui River". The god controlling long life "Great Fate" and the one with power over male offspring "Young Fate" were paid homage to as were the gods of the sun "Duke of the East", of the Yellow River "the Old Man of the River" and of the mountains "the Mountain Spirit". All of these votive songs referred to love. They are true love songs written with touching detail. "For Those Fallen for Their Country" is a hymn dedicated to heroes of the state of Wei. The description of these heroic figures in their struggle to the end with the enemy, their lack of fear at dying for a cause is written of in a stirring yet moving way. Finally the last section titled "The Last Sacrifice" describes the song and dance scene at the end of the ceremony. The beautiful young sorceresses carried fresh flowers which they handed from one to another as they sang and danced in turn. It would appear that votive song and dance in Chu, where shamanism enjoyed great popularity, had already attained a certain artistic level. Although ostensibly for the gratification of the gods, these rituals really provided entertainment for the spectators.

The popularity of folk song and dances produced many excellent artistes in the genre. It was already a means of livelihood for poor people then. "The Money-Makers", a chapter in the *Records of the Historian*, mentions people from the Kingdom of Zhongshan (part of the area of present-day Hebei Province). Many of them were driven by 'overcrowding and poor soil' to leave their homes and set out to earn their keep by working as actors or dancing girls. They would visit the women's quarters at the palace and the houses of feudal lords and nobles. Apart from playing musical instruments, the women also performed a quick stepped dance wearing heelless dancing shoes like slippers. The same book says that "Womenfolk from Zhao and Zheng" travelled long distances to make a living performing at rich people's houses. They played stringed instruments and excelled at dancing. Wearing long-sleeved dancing costumes and pointed dancing shoes without heels, they danced with expressive grace, sweeping up their long sleeves as they executed light dancing steps.

A feature of the Zhou "Dance of the People" was the sleeve movements. Many archaeological finds from the Warring States Period bear the figures of dancers swirling their sleeves. A Warring States ornament carved in jade in the form of two dancing girls unearthed at an old grave at Jincun in luoyang, Henan Province, serves as an example. The two dancers wearing long-sleeved dancing costumes which have full-length slim-waisted skirts. One of their hands is "with palm held upwards", the long sleeves flying above their heads, the other hand is "pressing with the palm", as their sleeves hang down brushing their hips. They are dancing together with spirited beauty (see fig. 8). A lacquered toilet case decorated with coloured drawings of dancing girls was unearthed at a Warring States tomb at Huangtuling in Changsha, Hunan. The dancing girls depicted are all clothed in long-sleeved, small-waisted dancing dresses. Three of them are busy practising a bending movement. One is an older woman with her sleeves rolled up and carrying a whip. Her expression is stern as if she is teaching them to dance or is coaching them. Another pair of people are standing between two pavilions, one of them has her arms held out slightly while the other is standing with them folded. The remaining five girls are probably resting after dancing (see fig.9). They are dancing girls in a rich family and are hard at work practising their dancing for the entertainment of the upper classes. The pot with banqueting, fishing, hunting and fighting designs unearthed in the Warring States tomb at Baihuatan in Chengdu, Sichuan, is inlaid with beautiful pictures. The middle band portrays the scene at a feast. In the top part of the hall

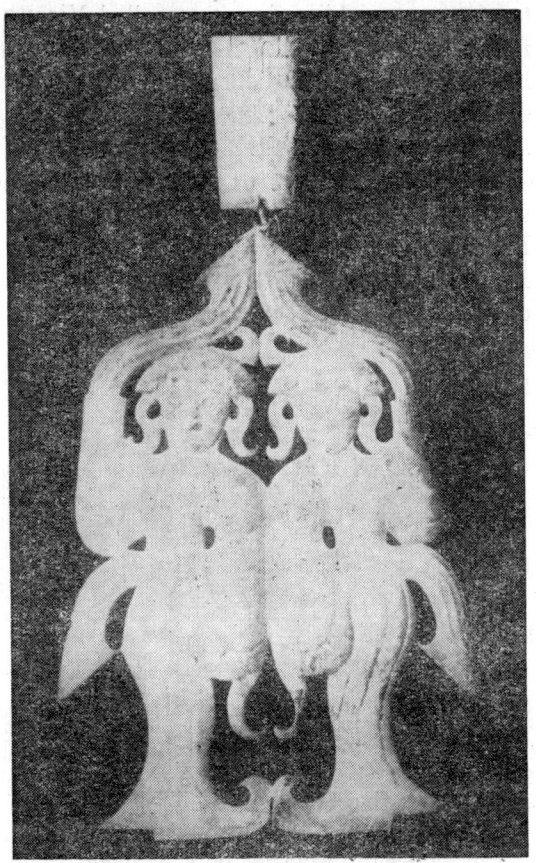

8. Warring States ornament of two dancing girls carved in jade. Unearthed at Luoyang, Henan.

the nobles are banqueting, at the bottom is a group dance scene. To the left hangs a string of bells. Beneath them the musicians are in mid performance. On the right hang some chime stones. Dancers clad in long-sleeved costumes with slim waists stand underneath. They are holding drumsticks in either hand as they twist and wave their arms as if beating the chime stone while dancing (see fig.10). Yet another pot with banqueting, fishing and hunting designs handed down from the Warring States Period, is decorated in basically the same way as the one from Baihuatan. Rubbings of details give a clearer view of the scene (see fig. 11). In the No.1 Eastern Zhou Tomb for people buried with the dead at Langjiazhuang in Linzi County, Shandong, figurines of dancing girls were found amongst the funerary objects. Their hairbuns are incomplete and their faces worn flat. Their eyebrows are painted in black and they are in graceful dancing poses, their long skirts brushing the ground as they lean to one side wriggling their waists (see fig. 12). Shandong Museum dates the grave from the late Spring and Autumn or early Warring States Period. Nine people buried with the dead have been discovered with an accompanying retinue of 17 others. The Academy of Sciences has identified them as young people from about 20 to 30 years of age. No doubt some were dancers.

Dancing girls were treated as mere objects for pleasure by the court and nobles during the war-torn Spring and Autumn and Warring States periods. In the tossle for power they were exchanged amongst the aristocrats or fell victim to their political struggles. According to the "Annals of Qin" in the *Records of the Historian*, Duke Mu of the Qin sent 28 dancing girls in 626 B.C.

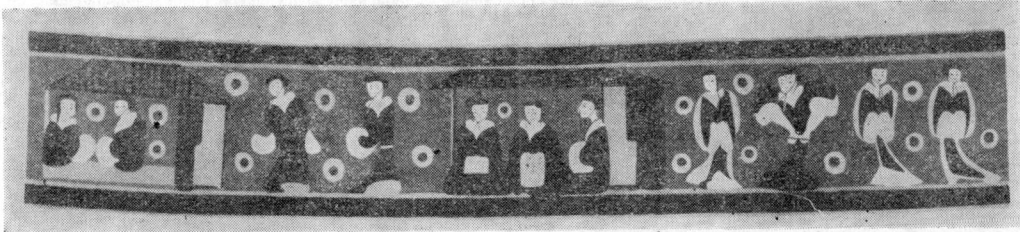

9. Copy of a Warring States lacquered toilet case decorated with coloured drawings of dancing girls. Unearthed at Changsha, Hunan.

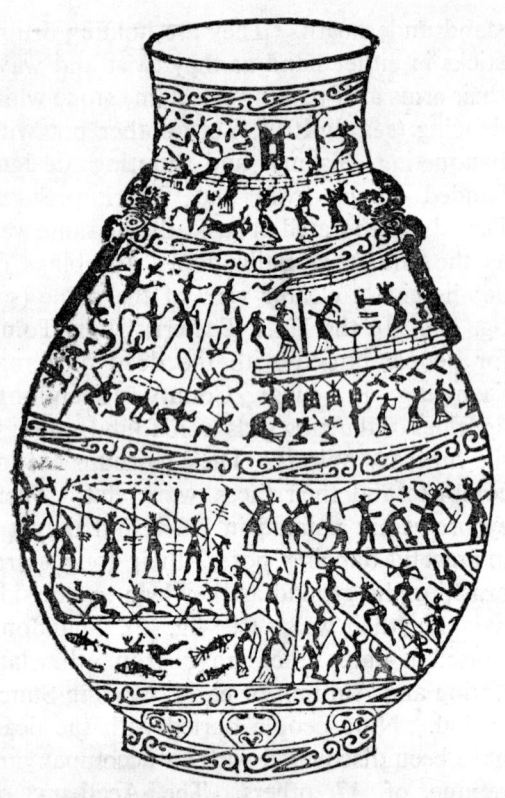

to a strong neighbouring state called Xirong in order to conquer it. The king there was led into a life of debauchery and was finally defeated by the Qin. *Zuoqiu Ming's Chronicles* states that in 562 B.C. the people of Zheng sent dancing girls and musical instruments as gifts to the Duke of Jin. "The Biography of Confucius" in *Records of the Historian* says that in 496 B.C. the state of Qi, afraid that Lu was becoming over-

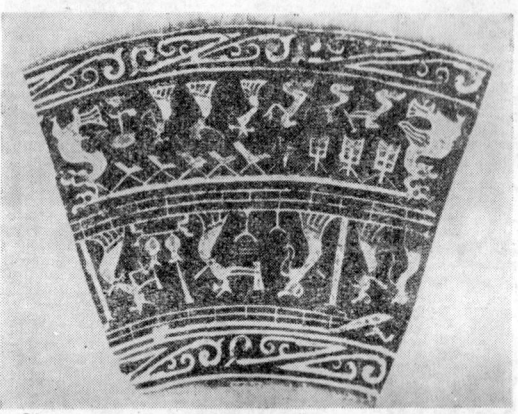

10. Copy of a Warring States pot with banqueting, music playing, fishing, hunting and fighting designs. Unearthed at Chengdu, Sichuan.

11. Warring States pot with banqueting, music playing, fishing and hunting designs. Rubbing of a section.

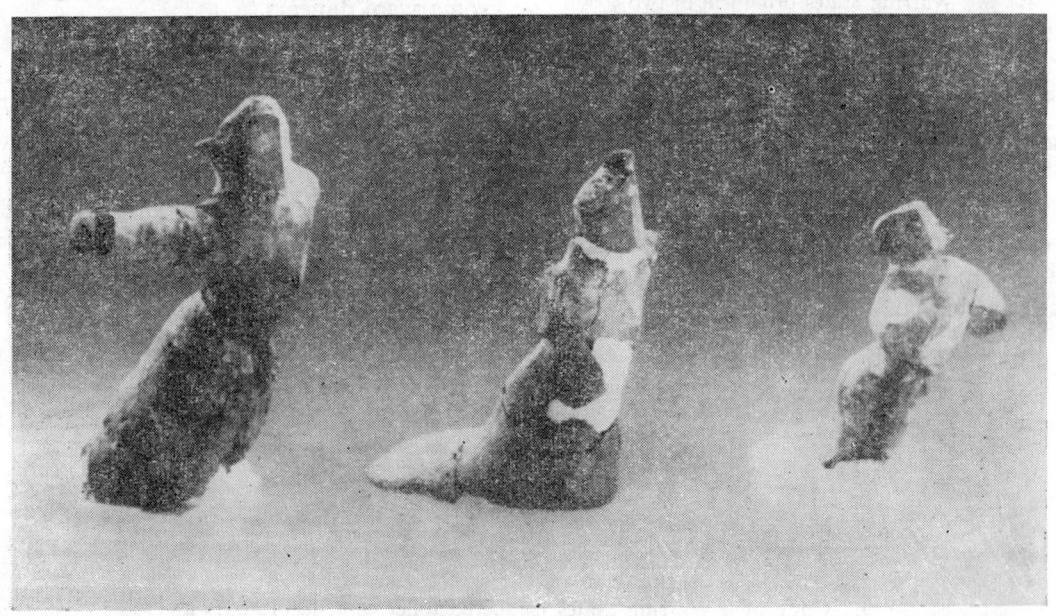

12. Eastern Zhou dancing figurines. Unearthed at Linzi, Shandong.

powerful, gave 80 beautiful women to its ruler, Ji Huanzi. They were dressed in bright clothes and danced the "Music from Kang", the name of a dance. From then on Ji Huanzi was so engrossed in this group of girls he neglected political affairs. The same book also says that in the spring of 500 B.C. Confucius went with Duke Ding of Lu to meet Duke Jing of Qi at Jiagu. A performance of "Music from the Palace" was given by artistes and dancers from the state of Qi. Angered, Confucius denounced them for being guilty of corrupting the feudal lords. They were killed on the spot. Thus, separated from their kinsmen, innocent performing artistes fell victim to the political struggles of the ruling class. Though they provided entertainment for the court and nobles, the song and dance performers remained in the position of slaves throughout the feudal period. They led hard lives, being bought and sold by others, given as presents or sentenced to death. Yet at the same time, due to the demands made on entertainment by the ruling class they acquired some of the conditions for improving the standard of their art. It was the output of this very group of professional song and dance artistes which spurred the development of dance in ancient China to a certain extent.

The flourishing of folk song and dance during the Spring and Autumn and Warring States periods and the creativity of song and dance artistes in various fields prepared the way for the development of "variety shows" and dance under the Han Dynasty.

CHAPTER FOUR

Han Dynasty "Variety Shows" and Dances

After a long period of military turmoil the First Emperor of Qin unified the six kingdoms in 221 B.C. and established the first multi-national centralized state to be dominated by the Han in the history of China. The brutal rule of the second Qin emperor was inundated by the rising tide of peasant revolts and the Han Dynasty (206 B.C.-A.D. 220) set up. During this period which marked the ascendancy of feudal power, the country was unified and the life of the people fairly stable. Economic progress and a powerfully rich state meant there were frequent contacts between different nationalities within the country as well as between China and other countries. Literature and art, including dance, thus developed to a new peak.

The establishment of a Board of Music in Qin and Han times gave a definite boost to the collection, sorting out and improvement of folk song and dance.

"Variety shows" were very popular during the Han. A string of all kinds of folk art such as acrobatics, martial arts, conjuring, comic performances, recitals of music, singing and dancing were included in a show. There were also more famous pieces such as "Duke Huang of the East Sea" and "The Gathering of Celestial Troupers".

They were a form of performing act which appealed to people. A book compiled by Huan Kuan during the Western Han (206 B.C.-A.D. 24) called *On Salt and Iron* mentions the popular acclaim for such shows. It goes on to say that the "actors and singing girls perform to an intricate arrangement of music". Moreover, "performers danced as elephants" at receptions for guests or as entertainment. Even when someone died song and dance and comic acts were performed. "Chronicle of the Emperor Wudi" in the *History of the Han Dynasty* states that "people came from 100 miles around to see acting performances in the spring of the third year of Yuanfeng [A.D. 108]." Following Zhang Qian's diplomatic mission to the Western Regions, music, dance and acrobatics from the area were introduced into the Central Plains (the middle and lower reaches of the Yellow River), thus enriching the contents of the "variety shows". At banquets of welcome for national minority or foreign guests, performances of "variety shows" on a grand scale were given. So clearly certain of the "variety shows" were representative of the standard of performing arts in the country.

Zhang Heng, a scientist and man of letters from the Eastern Han (A.D. 25-220) gives a fascinating description of the moving scene at a performance of a variety show at the Western Capital (present-day Xi'an in Shaanxi) in his *Rhyme-Prose on the Western Capital*. With the scenery set as a "Mountain of the Immortals" the show called "The

Gathering of Celestial Troupers" began. "Dancing Leopards and Bears" was a dance imitating the appearance and movements of various animals. The zither players were dressed up as "white tigers" and those on the bamboo wind instruments as "green dragons". Two actors in the parts of Ehuang and Nüying (said by legend to be the daughter of Yao and wife of Shun who later became the Goddess of the Xiangshui River and Lady of the Xiangshui River) sang in sweet clear voices. Hongya (supposed to have been a musician during the reign of the Three Emperors) directed, wearing a costume made of feathers. As the first item ended, "cloud and snow suddenly billowed forth". The snow fell increasingly heavily as "stones were turned to make thunder" (sound effects) everything shaking in the noise. Next, people dressed up as mythical creatures, big birds, white elephants and so on came on stage (performers in this kind of dance were called "elephant people") — a continuation of the tradition of "All the Animals Dance" from previous dynasties. A marvellous conjuring turn followed. "Strange shapes changed suddenly, things turned from one thing into another, there was sword swallowing and fire-breathing, everything was enveloped in smoke." The entire performance was an integrated series of acts — musical recitals, singing, animal dances and magic.

Further on, a performance of "Duke Huang of the East Sea" is described. Legend has it that Duke Huang from the East Sea had magic powers when he was young. He could ward off snakes and tigers. He wore a crimson band in his hair and an unsheathed sword at his belt. Towards the end of the Qin Dynasty, a white tiger was discovered near the East Sea. Duke Huang was asked to go and bring it under control. However he was getting old and drank too much so his magic powers did not work. As a result he did not subdue the tiger but was killed by it. This piece was included in "variety shows" during the Han Dynasty. It has a fixed plot and characters. It can be inferred that there was a fight between the man and tiger and equivalent performances of martial arts and dancing. Zhang Heng describes other acrobatic performances too, such as circuses and juggling or tight-rope walking and pole balancing.

"Variety show programmes" were not entirely the same but varied in scale.

Another performance at a reception for "tribal guests" is recorded in the "Record of the Western Regions" from the *History of the Han Dynasty*: "They were entertained with performances of the Bayu [name of a dance] Dulu [acrobatics and pole-climbing], Haizhong Dangji [name of a piece of music] and 'Endless Fish and Dragons' [a dance in fish and dragon costumes]." "Performances of the Bayu" were in fact the "Bayu Dances". "Chronicle of the Southern Tribes" in the *History of the Later Han Dynasty* says that the first emperor of the Han Dynasty, Liu Bang, launched an attack on the central Shaanxi plain area to put down three Qin generals who had betrayed him. He recruited some of the national minorities living in the area of Sichuan — the Cong — as soldiers. They were good, brave fighters and were also fond of singing and dancing. Liu Bang enjoyed the Cong folk songs and dances very much. He said they were songs from King Wu's defeat of King Zhou and ordered his minstrels to learn them. As the Cong lived in the Bayu area they were called "Bayu Dances". There were said to be four volumes of archaic words to go with the songs in the "Bayu Dances" but these could not be deciphered as they were probably a transliteration of the language of that nationality. In A.D. 222 under the Wei, the "Bayu Dances" were changed to "Zhaowu Dances" and during the Jin altered once again to "Xuanwu Dances", in both cases being used as ritual war dances. They were abolished in the Sui (A.D. 581-618) but included by the Tang in the "Music of Qingshang". The special quality of dances contained in that work was that "their contents should be refined, and the songs have style". Through being handed down at the Court over many years the "Bayu Dances" changed out of all recognition. However, the dances of the Cong must still preserve the original style as they have been carried on and developed within the nationality itself.

The large numbers of stone and brick reliefs as well as pottery figures unearthed in Han tombs provide a lifelike depiction of Han "variety shows" and dances in all their splendour.

The group of Western Han painted figurines of musicians, dancers and acrobats unearthed in the Western Han tomb at Wuyingshan, Jinan, Shandong Province, were moulded onto a clay tray. The figures on it are divided into two performing groups. On the left are the dancing girls wearing bright long-sleeved costumes tied with a sash. They are sweeping their long sleeves as they dance together. On the right, four of them are performing "handstands", "bending over" or doing "calithenics". Behind the dancers is the orchestra (see fig. 13). It is a realistic record of the various skills performed by song and dance artistes at banquets of the feudal aristocracy.

The "Picture of Variety Shows" on a Han stone relief from Yinan, Shandong is large and imposing. It gives a fairly full pictorial record of a variety show performance which includes acrobatics, horsemanship, bird and animal dances, the "Seven Tray Dance" and so on. But for the moment we will concentrate on a discussion of the dances. There is a full orchestra including percussion instruments such as bells, chime-stones and drums, wind instruments like reed-pipes with keyboards and flutes as well as different kinds of zithers in the stringed instrument section. Next to the drum decorated with coloured tassels and feather covers stands a man dressed in a wide-sleeved robe who is bending towards it. He has both arms raised about to hit the drum in a dancing pose full of vigour. In front of the orchestra a male dancer is performing the "Seven Tray Dance" famed in Han times. The seven trays are ranged along the ground in two rows with a drum in front of them. The dancer appears to be in the act of leaping off a tray — his right leg is "bending like a bow", while the left one is stretched out touching the ground with the foot near the drum. His body is upright as he looks back, the long sleeves of the dancing costume and band on his hat billowing out with the movement. He cuts a vigorous yet graceful figure (see fig.14).

There were various kinds of "Tray Drum Dances" during the Han for both male and female dancers. The number of trays and drums was variable so it is possible different arrangements were made according to the skill of the dancers. A Han brick relief from Pengxian County in Sichuan shows six trays spread on the ground with two drums placed between them. A woman dressed in a long-sleeved, slim-waisted dance costume is stepping on a drum in the "bending like a bow" pose. Her left hand stretches forwards, the long sleeve billowing while the right one is against her hip, its sleeve trailing behind in an elegant dancing posture (see fig.15). Although only a still-life stone carving it successfully depicts motion. The Han stone relief from the Wuban Tutelary Temple at Jiaxiang, Shandong, portrays a female dancer with both feet treading on a drum and swinging her hips. Another dancer is flinging the long decorated sleeves of her dancing dress upwards. The corners of her costume furl up in a lively stance of great beauty (see fig.16). The painted tower made of pottery unearthed at the Han tomb in Hewang Village, Xingyang, Henan Province, has a picture of song and dance on the front.

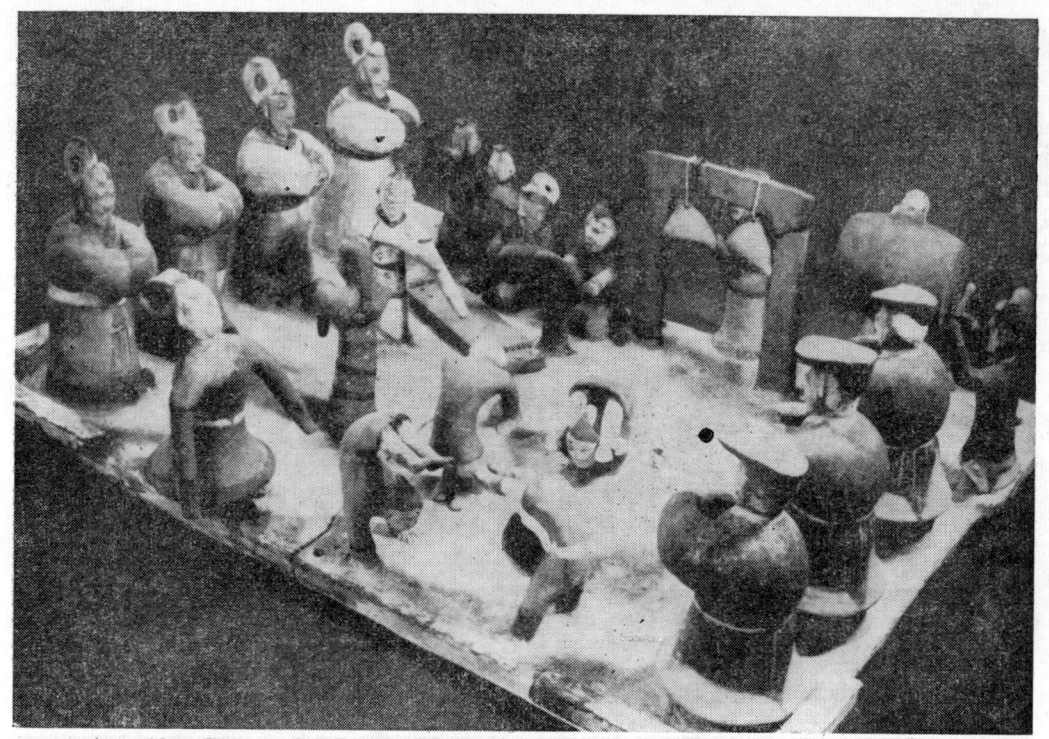

13. Group of Han clay figurines of musicians, dancers and acrobats. Unearthed at Jinan, Shandong.

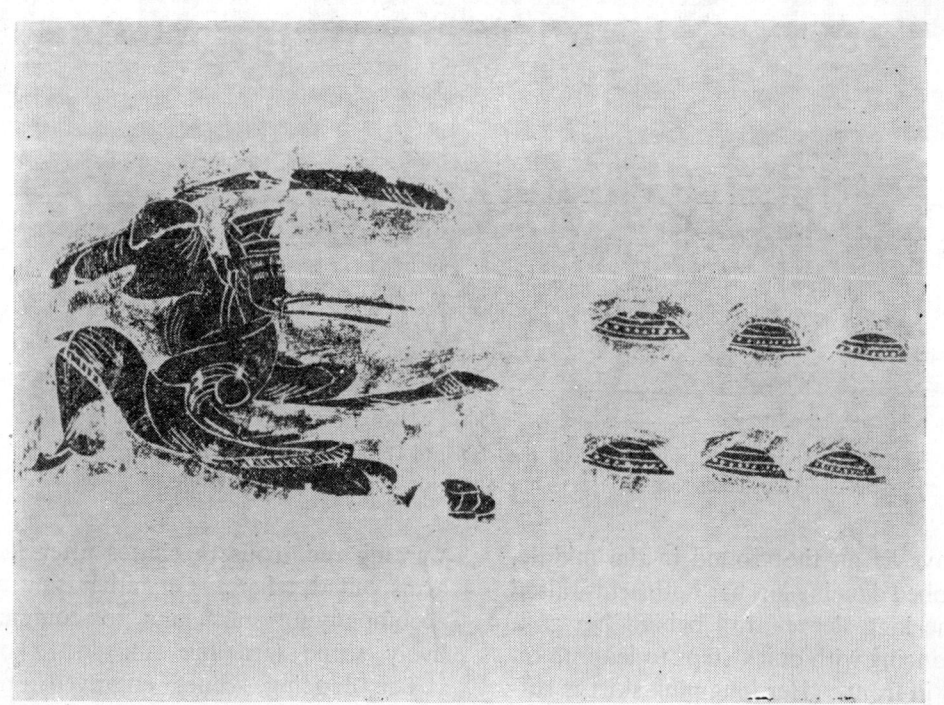

14. "Seven Tray Dance" from a Han stone relief of variety shows. Rubbing of a detail.

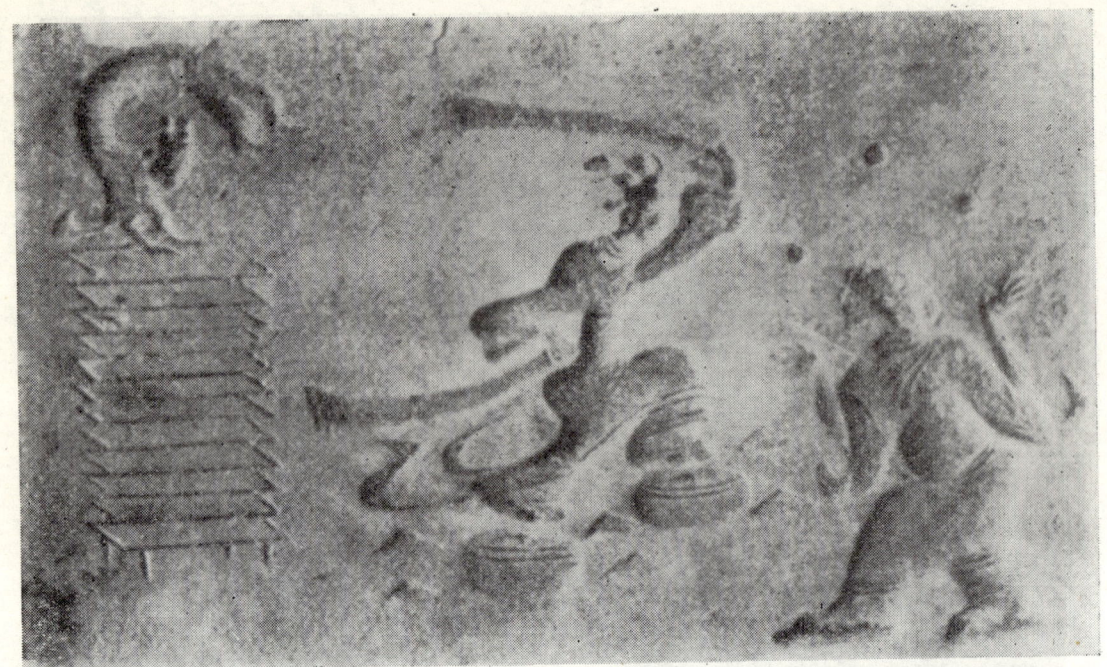

15. Han brick relief of "Tray Drum Dance" and acrobatics. Unearthed at Pengxian, Sichuan.

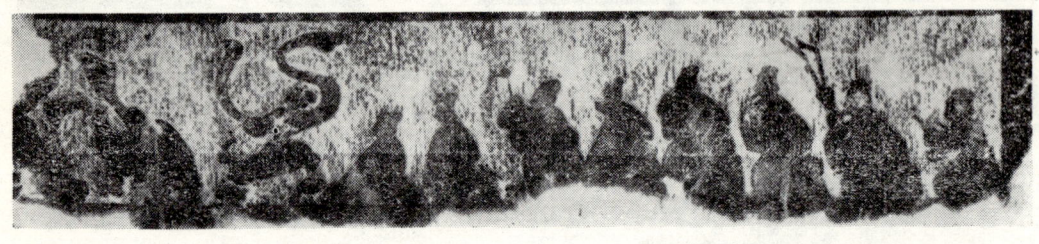

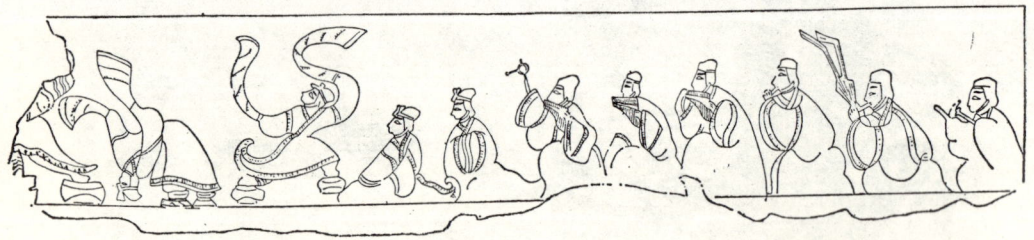

16. Rubbing and copy of the "Drum Dance" and accompanying musicians on an Eastern Han stone relief from Shandong.

Five trays lie on the ground in the middle. A red-robed dancing girl has both arms raised high, the long sleeves trail behind her as if she is dancing with quick steps to leap up on the tray in front. Her long pink skirt is ruffled up. Behind, a bare-chested dwarf wearing red trousers chases after her with arms outstretched. On either side are the accompanying musicians to complete the lively scene (see fig. 17).

The dancing scenes engraved on brick reliefs provide graphic corroboration of the

— 24 —

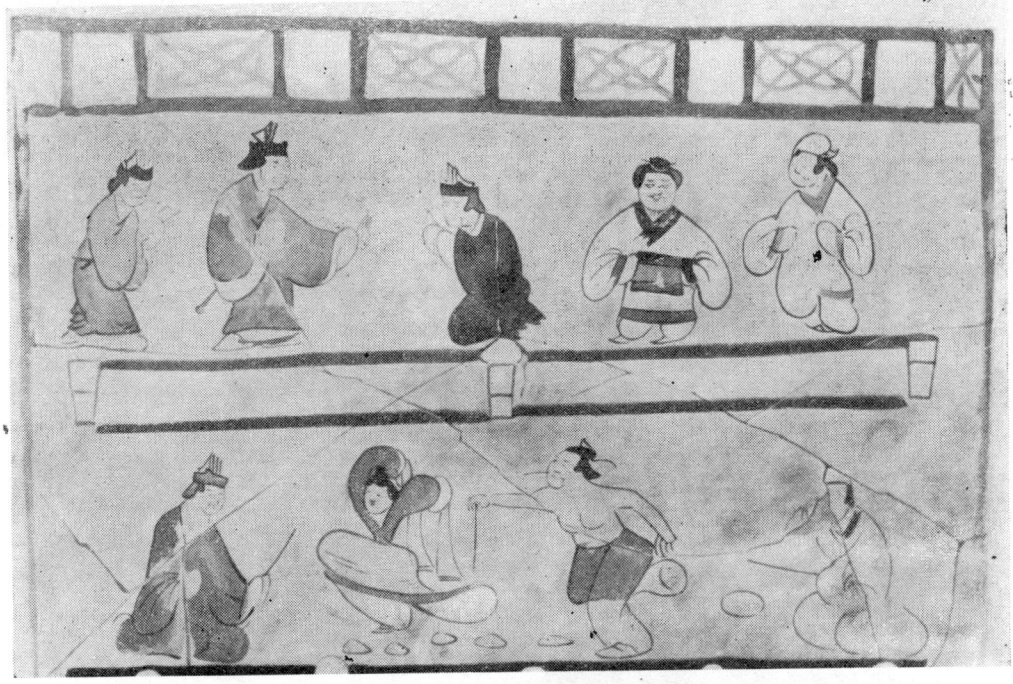

17. Copy of the picture of song and dance on the front of the Han painted earthenware tower. Unearthed at Yingyang, Henan.

spirited descriptions contained in the Han rhyme-prose. Zhang Heng in his *Rhyme-Prose on Dance* writes, "jump over seven trays and leap lightly", so dancers had to jump and step on the tray drums to make a rhythmic drumming sound as well as perform highly complex movements. In addition, they had to be energetic and supple and even more important have body control. If not, they would fail to meet his requirements for "jumping" high and lightly "leaping". Fu Yi's *Rhyme-Prose on Dance* says, "The rhythm for the treading is set by the drum.... Silk costume blows with the wind, long sleeves crossing over." The graceful and nimble movements made the sleeves and skirt of the dancing costume turn up. "When they turn back, the beat quickens, and they gently ascend, kneeling several times, walking on their insteps as they drop to brush the ground." As the musical accompaniment became quicker and quicker the dancer leapt and crouched to the rhythm, exactly as portrayed on the brick and stone reliefs described above. The "Tray Drum Dance" was an ingenious fusion of dance and acrobatics, a distinctive style in Chinese classical dance.

"Elephant people" acting in a show called "Endless Fish and Dragons" are also engraved on the stone relief of "variety shows" from Yinan, Shandong. The dragon, fish and peacock are behind the leader who is holding decorated fronds and a small hand drum with bead clappers. The dancers are ranged in a column dancing forwards. The "Fish Dance" which was one of the items (see fig. 18), resembled the "Carp Lantern Dance" still surviving as a folk tradition today. One dancer wears a fish costume with moving head and tail and wiggles them as if swimming along. He dances different patterns such as "Carp Leaping the Dragon Gate". The dragon and peacock in the stone

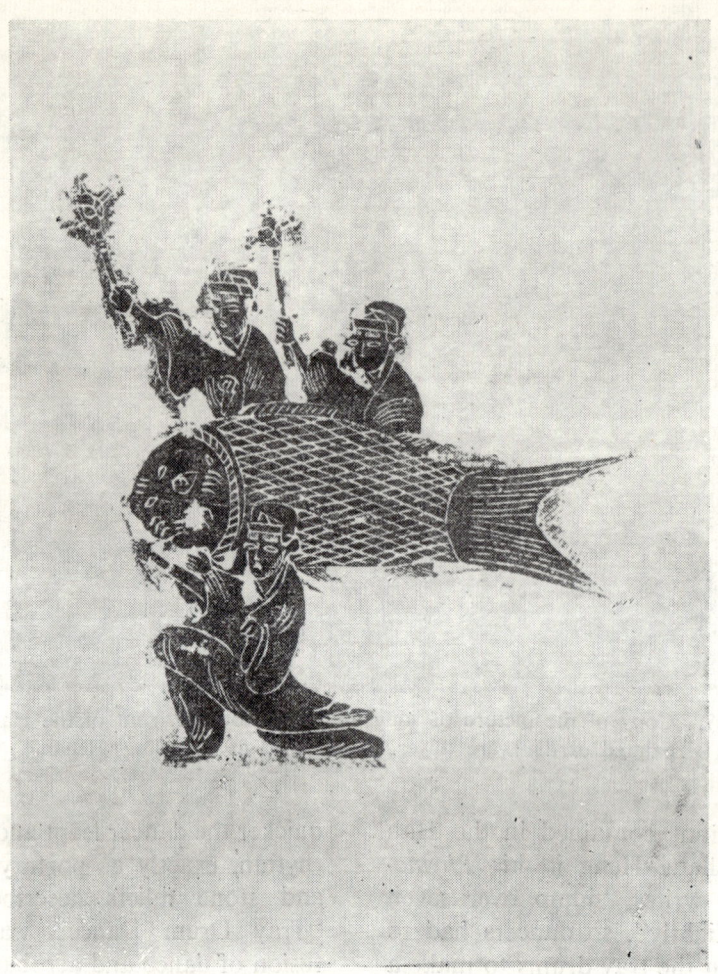

18. "Fish Dance" from a Han stone relief of variety shows. Rubbing of a detail.

engraving (see figs. 19 and 20) are wearing rather cumbersome costumes and props which, though very realistic, probably hampered their dance movements. Through the course of being handed down over the years, the skill with which these kinds of dances are portrayed has gradually improved and there are now more dance movements to depict the characteristics of the animals. The modern "Dragon Dance" uses an extremely light dragon prop and relies mainly on the performer to express the tossing and prancing of a giant dragon through his dancing. Another example is the "Peacock Dance" of the Dai nationality. In its original folk form, men performers danced, wearing a costume in the form of a peacock. After Liberation, dancers kept to the basic tradition but made some daring innovations. It was danced by female performers and the dress in the form of a peacock was no longer worn, there were just some designs symbolising the bird stitched onto the costume instead. Graceful choreography enabled the performers to give a lifelike portrayal of the beautiful gait of peacocks. One cannot fail to be moved at China's long and beautiful dance tradition on seeing stone reliefs over 2,000 years old being corroborated by contemporary folk dances as well.

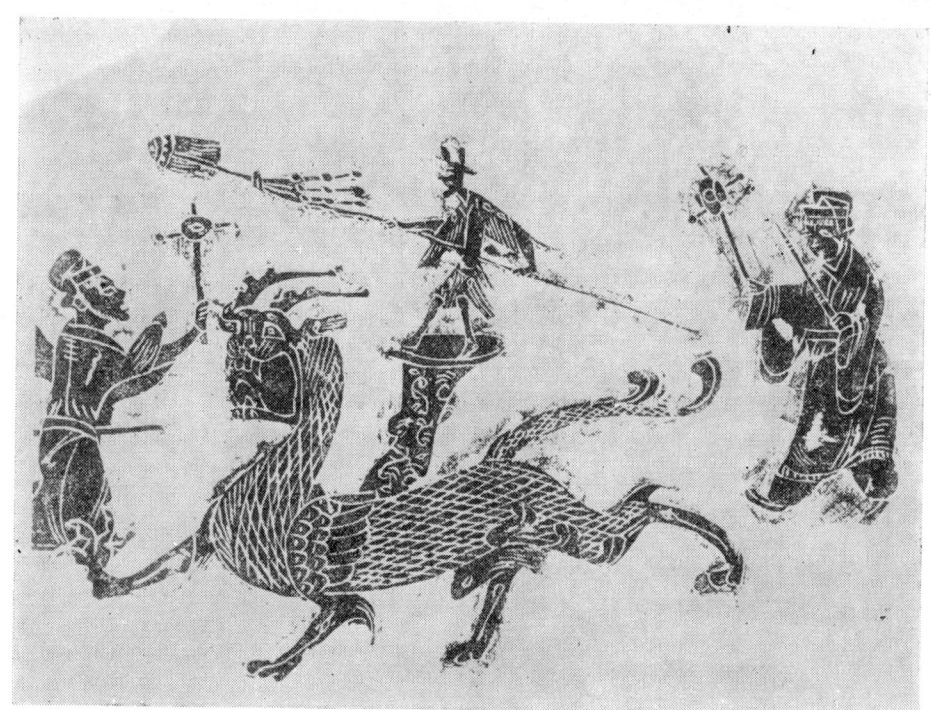
19. "Dragon Dance" from a Han stone relief of variety shows. Rubbing of a detail.

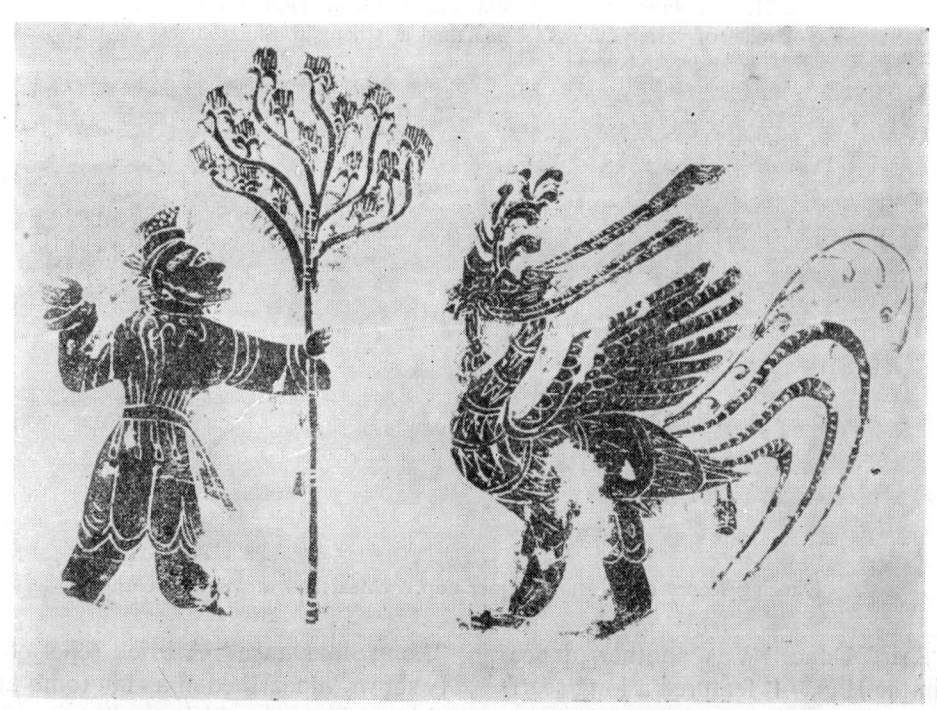
20. "Peacock Dance" on a Han stone relief of variety shows. Rubbing of a detail.

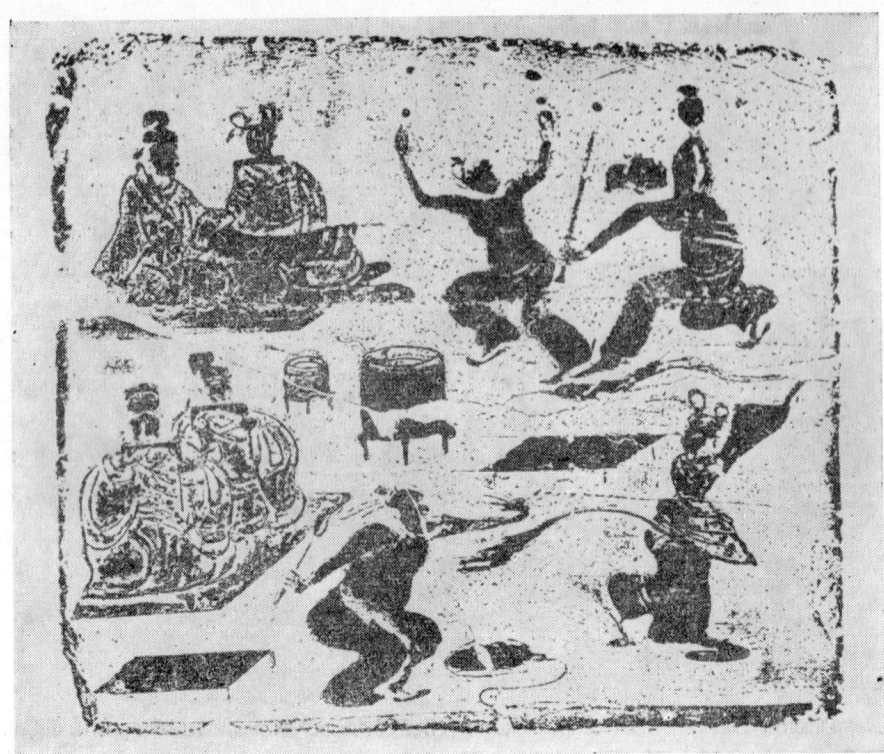
21. Rubbing of song and dance on a Han brick relief of variety shows. Unearthed at Chengdu, Sichuan.

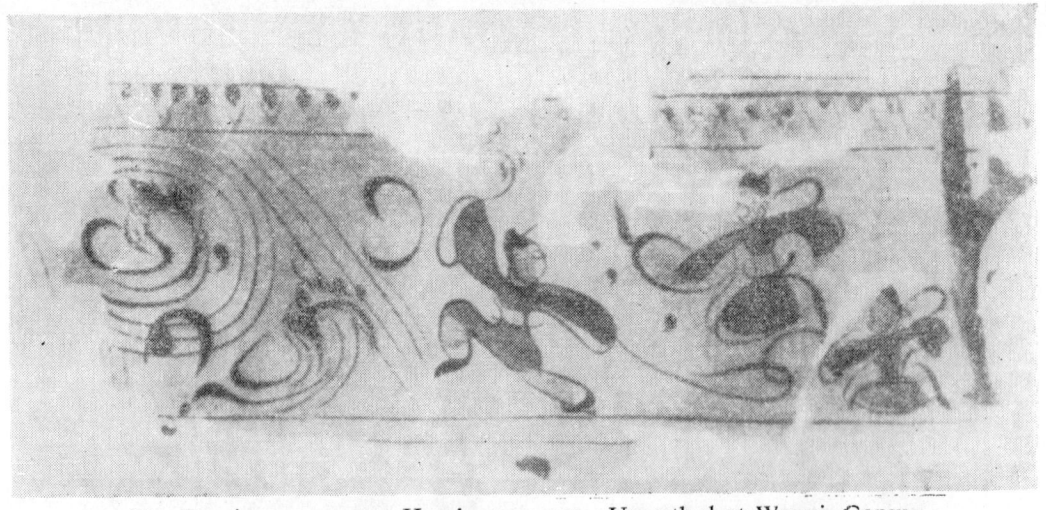
22. Dancing scenes on a Han lacquer cup. Unearthed at Wuwei, Gansu.

The "Scarf Dance" was another dance famous in the Han. It featured a long scarf which was held in both hands during the dance — very similar to the present day "Long Silk Dance". A brick relief of "variety shows" unearthed at a Han tomb at Yangzishan, Chengdu, Sichuan Province, depicts a dancing girl, her hair worn in two coils, clad in a short costume and long pair of trousers with embroidered edges. She is holding a long piece of silk in a dancing pose similar to "Shooting Wild Geese". It floats sideways in the air, a short rod wrapped in the silk clearly visible amongst the ends she is holding. By dancing this way, less effort is needed and the execution of fairly difficult movements is made easier. Behind the dancing girl is a funny man, who carries a drum and is holding out his arms as he moves squatting across the ground as if chasing the girl. The role was probably played by a dwarf and the like (see fig. 21).

Pictures of dancing are painted on a lacquer cup uncovered at the Mozizui Han tomb in Wuwei, Gansu. A long ribbon billows out between the hands of a dancer as

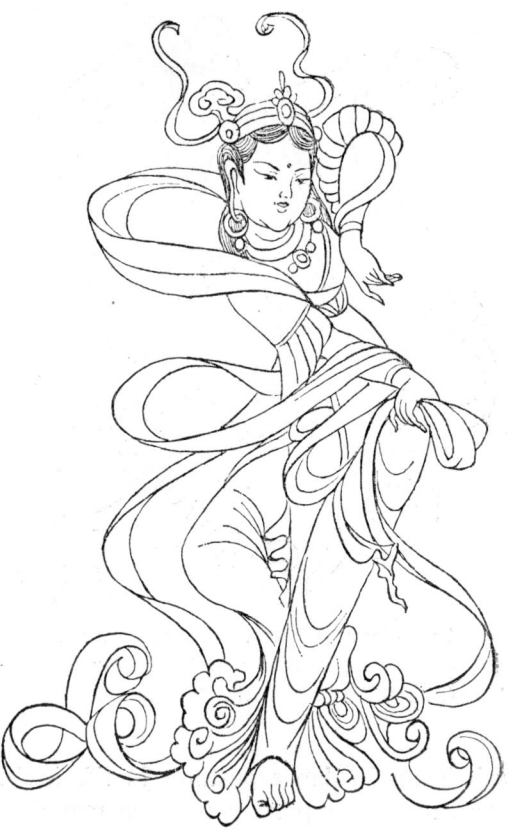

24. Copy of part of the dance on a High Tang mural from Dunhuang at Cavern No. 148 in the Mogao Caves.

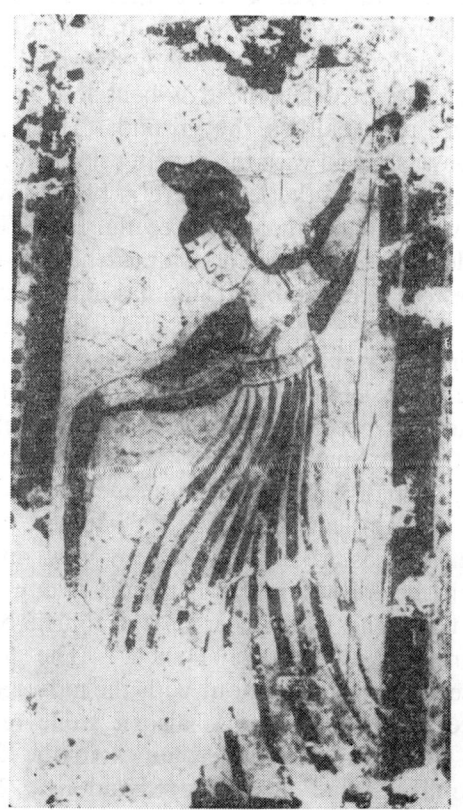

23. Tang mural of a red costumed dancing girl. Unearthed at Xi'an, Shaanxi.

in the dances with scarves (see fig. 22) which are a folk tradition in China.

A mural of a red-costumed dancing girl from the Tang (A.D. 658) was discovered in an old tomb in Xi'an, Shaanxi. Wearing a short costume with a long, pleated skirt, the dancer, her hair in a tall bun, has a long shawl draped over her shoulders. The shawl is stretched out in an oblique line by her arms in a beautiful dancing pose (see fig. 23). In certain religious pictures, like the figures of celestial entertainers and flying celestials, dance poses with long silk scarves trailing out are depicted (see figs. 24 and 25). Such poses are removed from real life, being mainly for decorative effect. However, the artists must have found the inspiration to portray

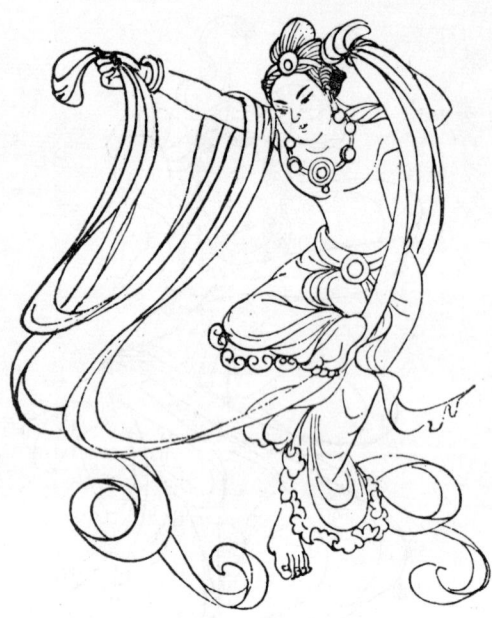

25. Copy of part of the dance on a High Tang mural from Dunhuang at Cavern No. 180 in the Mogao Caves.

such beautiful dance postures in life itself. These too are important research materials for the study of the ancient "Scarf Dance". The form of the dance has been preserved all along in both folk and Chinese opera dances. After Liberation, dancers created the fiery "Red Silk Dance" and beautiful "Long Silk Dance", with its many poses, from these traditional dances. The late dramatist Ouyang Yuqian once said that opera artists (playing female roles) of the late Qing created a type of silk dance. The silk was more than seven metres long. At the very height of the dance the dancer would suddenly give a flick and the long silk would flow from his hands, float right round above the heads of the audience to be retrieved by the performer who then continued the dance. This really calls for a very high degree of dancing skill. Perhaps in the future some dancers, while keeping to the tradition, can improve their performing ability enough to bring back this dance manoeuvre which has been lost to the stage.

The *Miscellaneous Records of the Western Capital* states that "Qi, companion to the Han Emperor Gaodi, is an excellent drum, zither and lute player. She is also good at dances in which the sleeves are turned up and waist bent." The phrase 'sleeves turned up and waist bent' does not appear to be a dance term but a general name for a kind of dance characterized by special sleeve actions and bending movements. As mentioned before, these sleeve movements are an ancient tradition in China. Depictions of the tossing of sleeves abound on Han brick reliefs. Sleeves came in many different forms. One was a long, narrow sleeve equal in width at top and bottom (similar in style to the long sleeves in Tibetan dance). An example is on an early Han brick relief from Nanyang in Henan. With her hair up in a high bun, the dancer is dressed in a long-sleeved dancing costume. Her head is bent low as she gazes at a ball on the ground. Her right elbow is raised with the dancing sleeve hanging down and the left sleeve is being swept downwards at an angle (see fig. 26). The jade carving of a dancer unearthed at the Western Han tomb at Dabaotai in the Fengtai District of Beijing (Peking) is in a long skirt, the right hand is held high as it flicks the long sleeve which coils behind her in a beautiful pose (see fig. 27). A stone relief at Qufu in Shandong portrays a dancer wearing a small hat (or head ornament) dressed in a long-sleeved coloured costume. Her general posture makes it seem very much as if she is leaping with her arms swung out in front and behind her on the fourth beat during the "Yangge Dance". The long sleeves are billowing out with the movement (see fig. 28). There is also a stone relief of song, dance and acrobatics in the Dai Family Shrine at Qufu, Shandong. The dancing girl in the picture is wearing the same kind of long, narrow-sleeved dancing costume (see fig. 29) too.

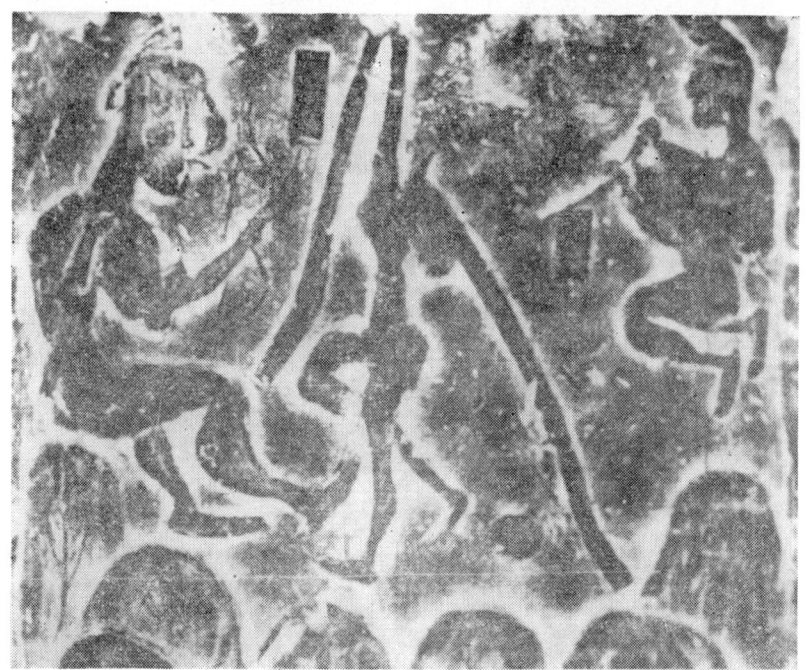

26. Rubbing from a Western Han brick relief of song and dance. Unearthed at Nanyang, Henan.

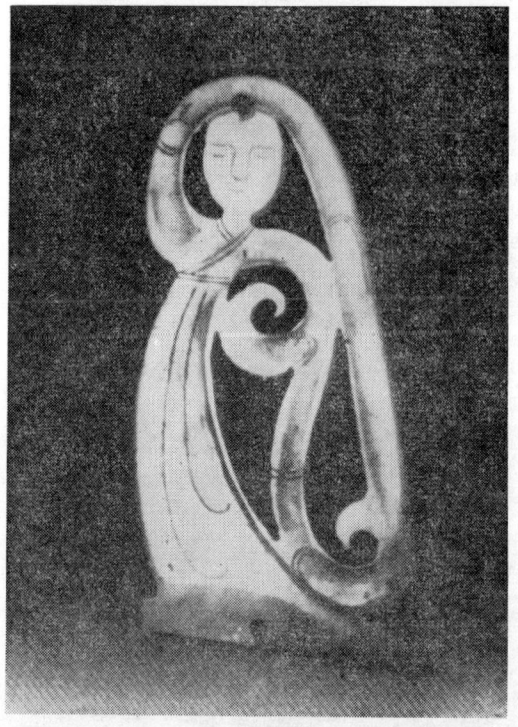

27. Western Han jade carving of a dancer. Unearthed at Beijing.

There was another kind of Han dancing sleeve which was wide and long. The clay figures of dancers, one with her sleeves swept back and another making a greeting gesture with cupped hands uncovered at a Western Han tomb in Xi'an are examples where this kind of clothing is worn (see fig. 30). On the figurine with sleeves flicked back the long left-hand sleeve has been worn away but the one for the right hand is swept across the shoulder to hang down the back. She has a gentle expression (see figs. 31 and 32).

One other type was a slim-waisted long-skirted robe with broad arms which extended in a long, narrow sleeve at the wrist like the "water sleeves" in Chinese opera costumes. For example, there are the richly dressed clay dance figurines unearthed from an Eastern Han tomb in the eastern suburbs of Guangzhou in the "throwing back the shoulders, palms pressing downwards" dancing pose (see fig. 33). There are two dancers on a Han stone relief from Tengxian

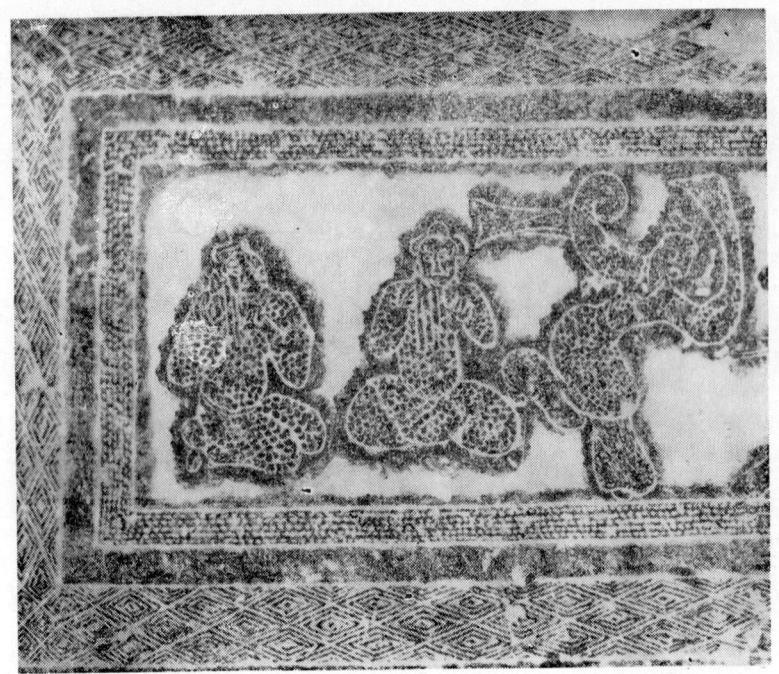

28. Rubbing from a Han stone relief of song and dance from Qufu, Shandong.

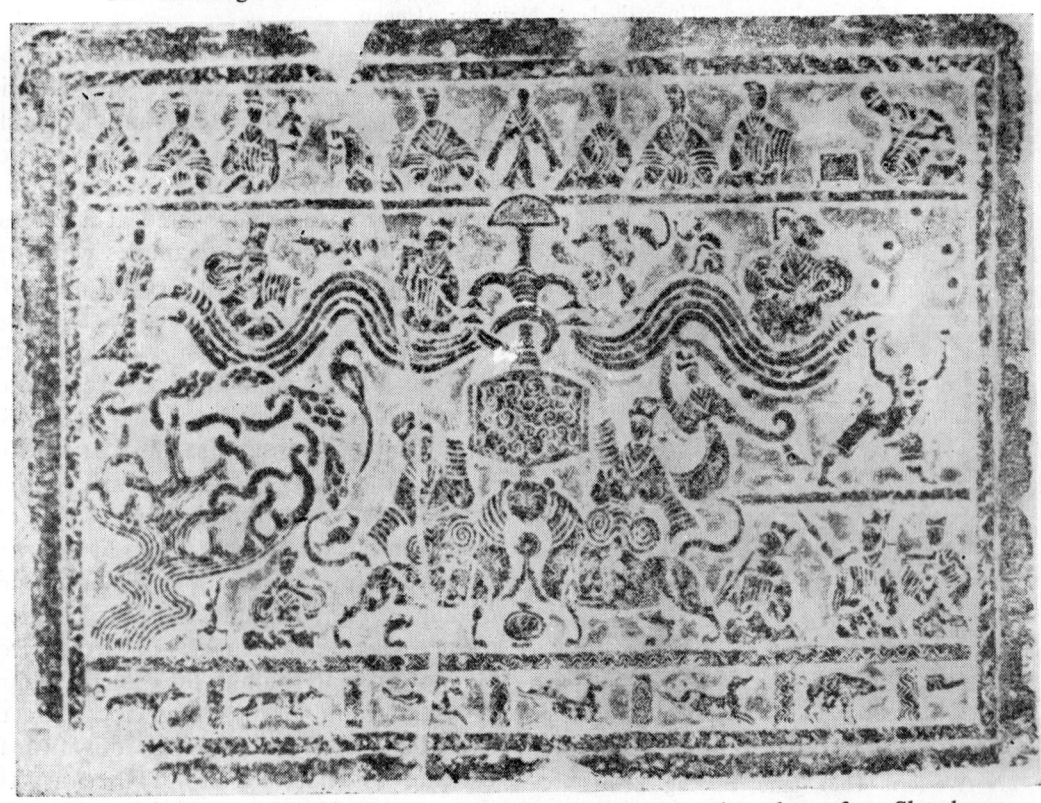

29. Rubbing of song and dance from a Han stone relief of variety shows from Shandong.

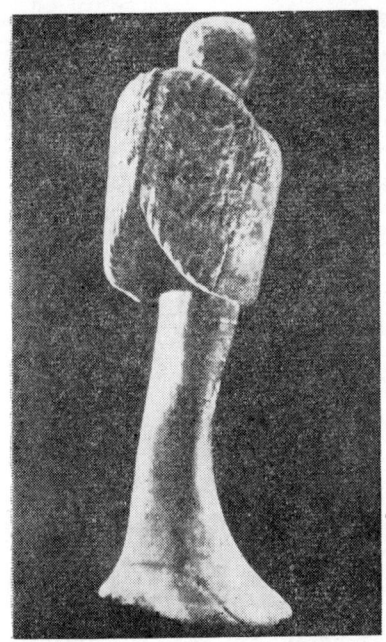

30. Han figurine of a dancer cupping her hands in greeting. Unearthed at Xi'an, Shaanxi.

County in Shandong both wearing hats and trailing their long sleeves as they dance facing each other (see fig. 34). Dancers depicted on a Han stone relief from Liucheng in Jiangsu are on a low couch. They are twisting up their long sleeves as they dance (see fig. 35). The silk picture discovered at the Han tomb at Jinqueshan in Linyi, Shandong, has a dancer sweeping her sleeves back as she performs (see fig. 36). The Tian family bronze mirror of carters uncovered at a Han tomb in Shaoxing, Zhejiang, shows a slim dancing girl in a long skirt gracefully holding her arms in a pose similar to the "flag blowing in the wind". Her sleeves billow in a beautiful dancing posture (see fig. 37). The clay figure of a dancing girl from the Han tomb at Tianhuishan, Chengdu in Sichuan is lifting her skirt with her left hand while her right hand is raised slightly in a gentle dancing posture (see fig. 38). All of the dancing figures described above have the same kind of long, narrow dancing sleeves project-

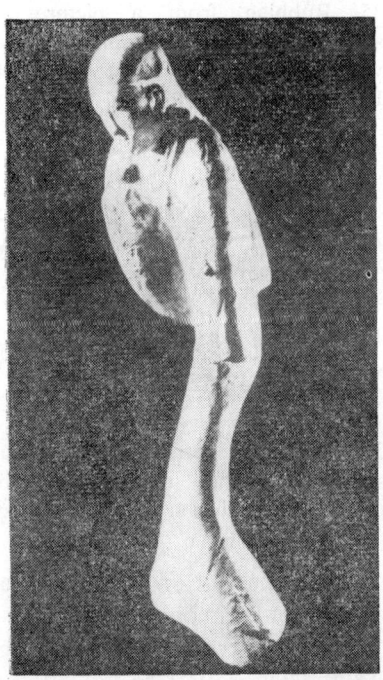

31. Side view of a Han figurine of a dancer with a sleeve swept back. Unearthed at Xi'an, Shaanxi.

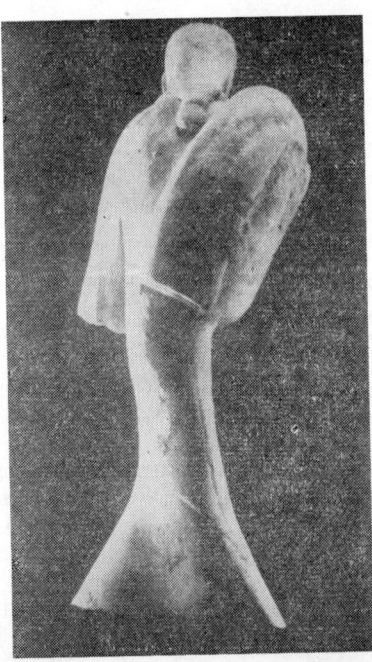

32. Back view of the Han figurine of a dancer with a sleeve swept back.

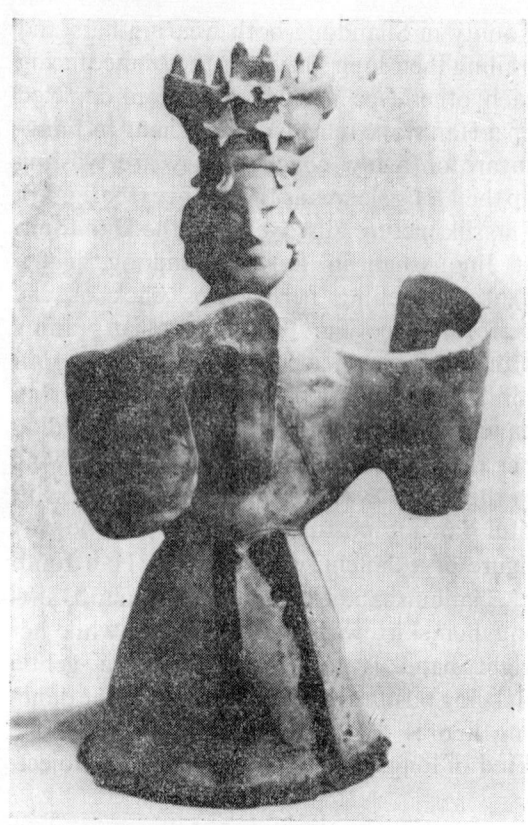

33. Han painted figurine of a dancing girl. Unearthed in the eastern suburbs of Guangzhou.

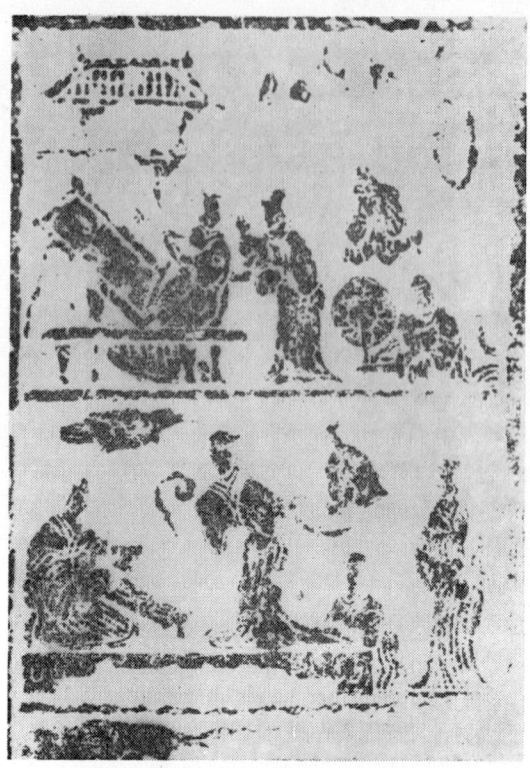

35. Rubbing from a picture of song and dance and spinning and weaving on a Han stone relief. Unearthed at Peixian, Jiangsu.

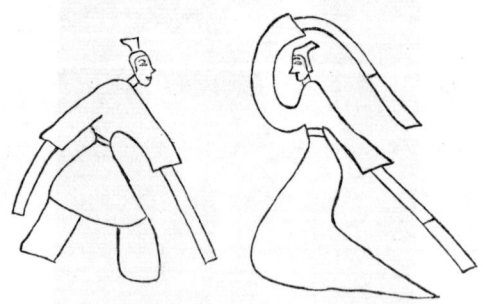

34. Copy of a detail from a Han stone relief of a man and woman dancing together from Tengxian, Shandong.

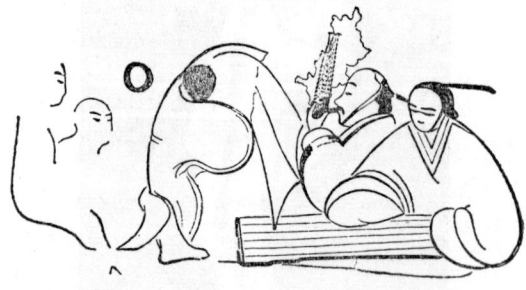

36. Copy of an illustration of song and dance on a Han silk picture. Unearthed at Linyi, Shandong.

ing from their broad-armed costumes. Dancers on the stone relief of the Drum Dance from Qufu in Shandong are wearing long-sleeved dancing costumes as well.

Drumsticks poke out from their sleeves as they dance together in pairs striking the drum. Their "bow and arrow" step dancing pose is strong and vigorous (see fig. 39).

There is an abundance of material on the history of dance in the Han Dynasty,

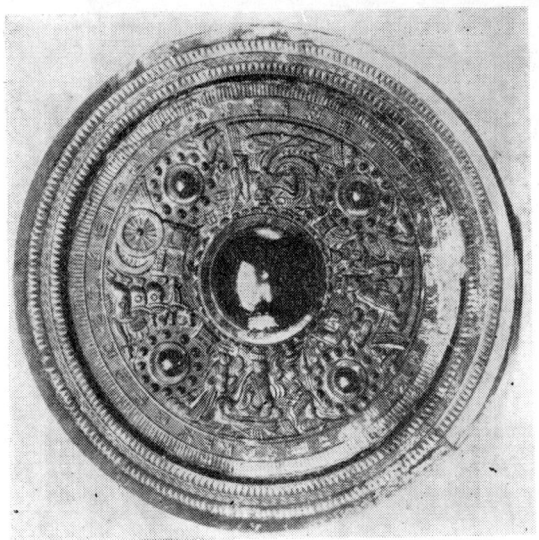 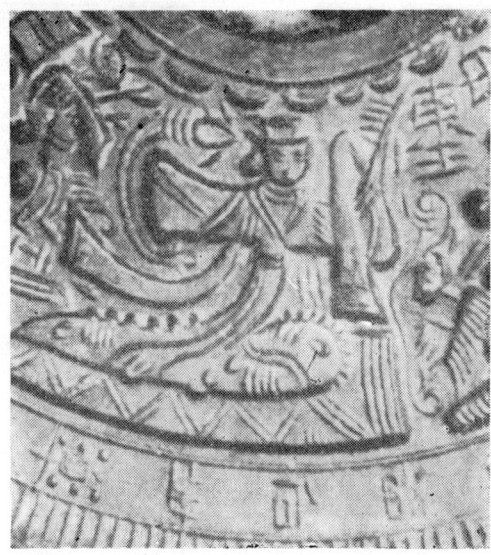

37. The Tian family mirror of carriage and human figures, and detail of a dancer. Unearthed at Shaoxing, Zhejiang.

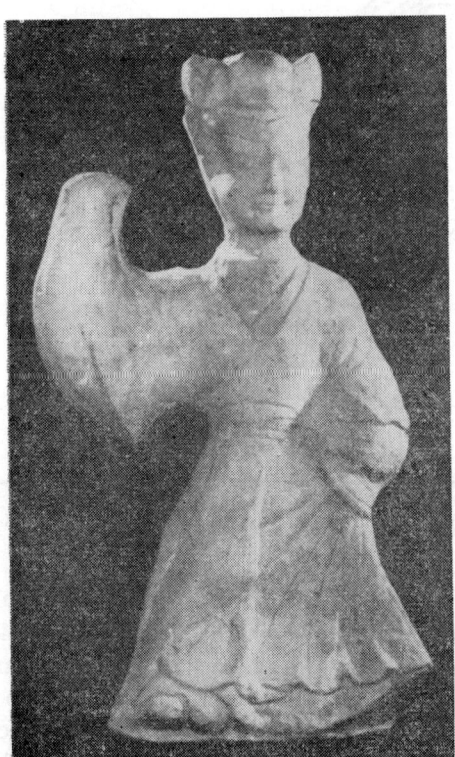

38. Han figurine of a dancing girl. Unearthed at Chengdu, Sichuan.

especially representational materials. During the period of more than four hundred years that the Eastern and Western Han lasted, various professional and amateur dancers created many gorgeous dances through their own hard work. However, as song and dance artists were looked down on there are few traces of their names in historical records. The figurines of dancers and stone engravings of song and dance "variety shows" were burial articles for the feudal nobles. They were under the illusion that after dying they would go to another world where they could continue ordering the singers and dancers to entertain them. For this reason funerary objects were interred in their burial chambers. However, this serves to provide us with a large body of realistic yet lively material on the history of dance. As for literary records, often it is only by some coincidence, such as one particular dancer being favoured by a top feudal ruler that their life and art are described in the history books. This does enable us to find out something about the development of ancient dance.

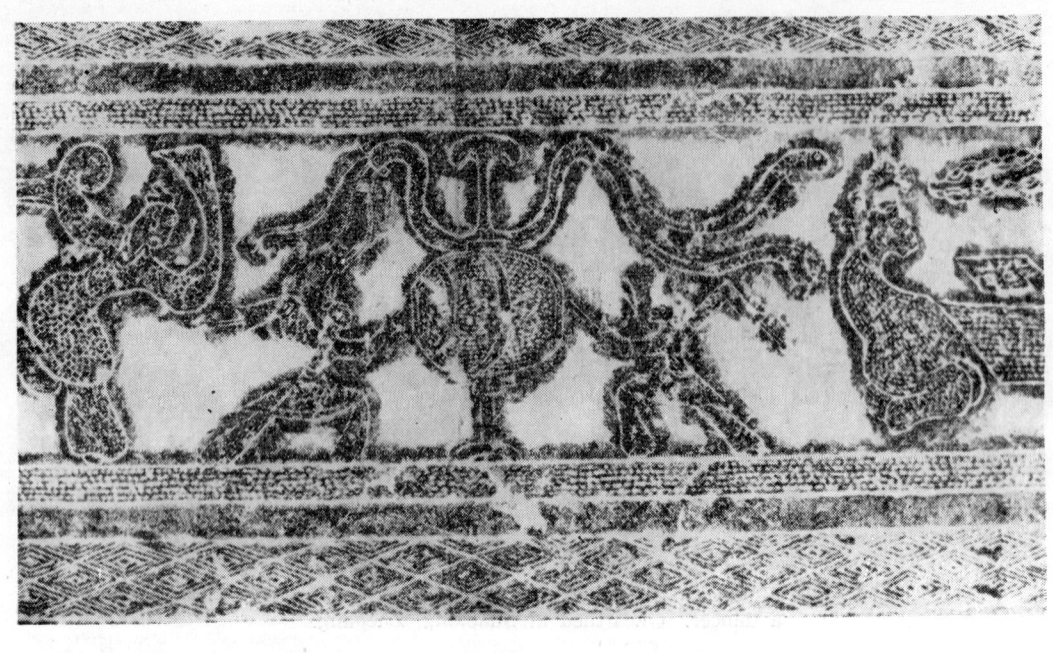

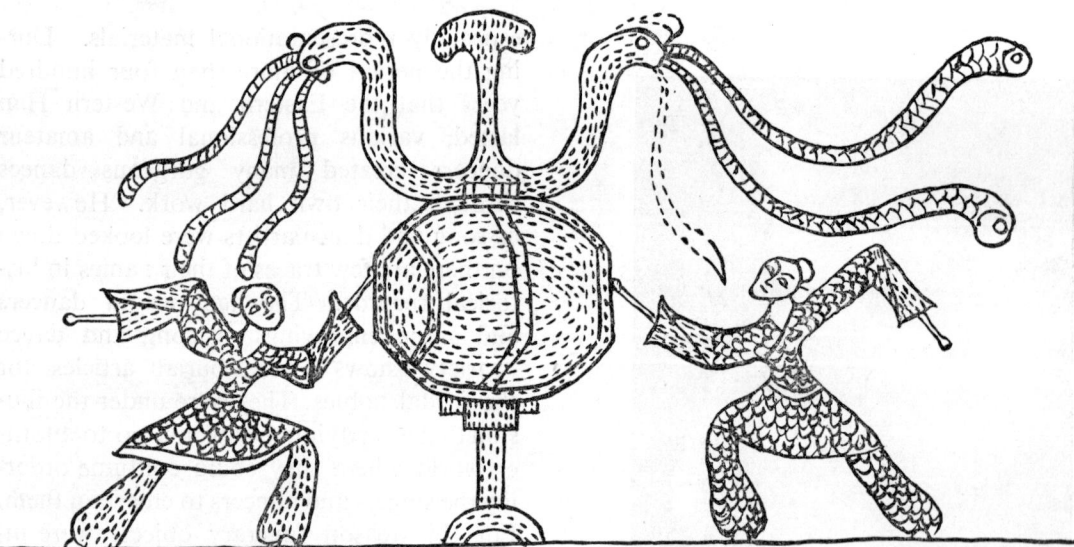

39. Rubbing and copy of a picture of the "Drum Dance" on a Han stone relief from Qufu, Shandong.

A girl living during the Han called Zhao Feiyan was supposed to have been as light as a swallow. She was a skilled singer and dancer so was called "Flying Swallow" (Feiyan). Feiyan's father died when she was young and she was left homeless. She ended up at the capital city, then Changan, later acting as serving-girl to the household of Princess Yang's where she studied singing and dancing. Feiyan worked extremely hard and would often forget to eat so absorbed was she in her study of the art of dance. She was good at breath control, had a light, graceful dancing gait and outstanding technique. "She excelled at light steps" floating like a flowered branch held in someone's hand, probably a reference to a deft kind of quick, short step. Later, she was taken into the palace by the Emperor Chengdi and received the title of Jieyu which denoted a particularly accomplished concubine. Subsequently she was made Empress. However, on the Emperor Chengdi's death, Aidi took the throne but soon died as well. Finally, when the next emperor, Pingdi, came to power Feiyan was demoted to an ordinary citizen and ordered to commit suicide.

The life of Wang Wengxu also shows us how singers and dancers were trained as well as the tragic way in which girls from ordinary backgrounds were abducted and ended up as song and dance artists. At the age of eight or nine Wengxu was entrusted to the care of the Liu Zhongqing household where she studied song and dance. Four or five years later when Wengxu went home she told her mother that Jia from Handan had come looking for song and dance girls and that Liu Zhongqing wanted to give her to him. Wengxu's mother immediately took her away to the safety of her grandmother's house. Liu Zhongqing and Wengxu's father found them. Anxious and scared, Wengxu's mother said that although her daughter had been living at Liu Zhongqing's house they had not asked for any money and so had not sold her. So why did he want to give the child away? Liu Zhongqing slyly denied that he would ever do so. But just a few days after she returned to his house Wengxu rode past her own home in Jia's carriage and cried "They are indeed taking me away. We're going to Liusu!" Her father and mother rushed to Liusu and saw Wengxu. They all burst into tears. Wengxu's mother said she was going to lodge a complaint but her daughter persuaded her that it was not necessary as it was at least somewhere to stay so what was the point of going to the Law. Subsequently Wengxu's parents followed her to Lunu in Zhongshan and found their daughter staying with five other entertainers. They tried repeatedly to get their daughter back but failed as the father was penniless. They were forced to let their daughter be taken away by other people. From then on, Wengxu lost touch with her family. After going to Jia's house in Handan, she was sent at the age of 20 to Prince Wei's household in Chang'an as a domestic entertainer. In 91 B.C. Wengxu bore a child called Liu Xun by Prince Wei's son, Shi. Later the whole household was killed including Wengxu but her son Liu Xun survived to become emperor, that is the Han Emperor Xuandi. This was the only reason that Wengxu's life was recorded in history books.

Another Han emperor, Liu Bang, doted on his concubine Qi who was expert at 'Dancing throwing up her sleeves and bending at the waist' and dances from the area of Chu. She could also play the zither and sing. Liu Bang wanted to depose the son of the Empress Lü and set up Qi's son as prince. However the Court ministers were against it. After Liu Bang's death, the Empress Lü had Qi imprisoned in the Palace gaol. She was ordered to wear convict's clothes, had her hair shaved off and was made to hull grain. She sang sadly that "The son has become prince but his mother is a prisoner, all day long I hull grain until evening, often with Death as a companion, separated by so many miles, who can I send to tell you?" When the Empress Lü heard this she was very angry and had Qi's son summarily killed. Qi's hands and feet were broken, her eyes gouged out and her ears singed. She was forced to drink some medicine that made her mute, was flung into the toilet and called " Human Pig".

The three people described above were just those who by chance reached the highest levels of feudal government out of the vast numbers of song and dance artistes.

These accounts tell us two things about the state of affairs then. Firstly, dancers in the Han Dynasty already had to undergo strict, professional training from an early age. The art of dance had reached a fairly high standard so there were skills such as bending movements, sleeve actions and special dance steps. They were also already aware of the need for good breath control to enable the waist and limbs to attain the strength and suppleness required for a graceful dancing posture. Secondly, song and dance artistes were of a low social status and only by chance became the fancy things of the highest feudal rulers. Though they then enjoyed a high position, they were weak and powerless within the ruling group due to their impoverished backgrounds. Thus struggle as they might they could not escape their tragic end.

It was the self same song and dance artistes, "variety show" performers and ethnic folk dancers that were looked down upon by the feudal ruling class who through their combined efforts raised dance during the Han Dynasty to a new level.

CHAPTER FIVE

The Exchange of Song and Dance Between Different Nationalities

At the end of the Eastern Han a situation emerged in which the three Kingdoms of Wei, Shu and Wu were in a three sided confrontation. Not long after the Western Jin (A.D. 265-316) defeated the Wu and unified China, there began yet another unsettled period torn by war. With the move southwards of the political centre of the Han people then, minority nationalities in large numbers poured into the Central Plains leading to antagonisms at different times between the Eastern Jin (A.D. 317-420) and Sixteen Kingdoms (A.D. 304-439) as well as between the Southern Dynasties (Song, Qi, Liang, Chen) (A.D. 420-589) and the Northern Dynasties (Nothern Wei, Eastern Wei, Western Wei, Northern Qi, Northern Zhou), (A.D. 386-581). However the migration and intermingling of peoples meant that there was a constant exchange of culture giving rise to a period in which music and dances were transmitted between different nationalities.

Following the move into Central China of minority nationalities from the Northwest much of the music and dance from their areas as well as from abroad was brought to the Central Plains. An example is those from Kucina (now the area of Kucha in Xinjiang) which were fairly influential and probably introduced in A.D. 384. Kucina had always been a fertile area for folk song and dance. The Tang monk Xuanzang's *Records of the Western Regions of the Great Tang Dynasty* says "the kingdom of Quzhi [i.e. Kucina] ... has an ordered air and is rich in customs. ... For musical arts it is the best of all the kingdoms." After they were brought to the Central Plains Kucina music and dance became very popular. Perhaps the reason was its lively melody, distinct rhythm and the fact that it was highly suitable as a dance accompaniment. As a result "Kucina music" was employed in many dances of the Northern Zhou (A.D. 557-581) and Sui and Tang dynasties. In addition, there was also music and dance from Shule (the area of present day Kashi and Shule in Xinjiang) and Bokhara (now the area of Bukhara in the Uzbek Soviet Socialist Republic) which were introduced into the Central Plains in A.D. 436 when the Emperor Taiwu of the Northern Wei established contact with the Western Regions. In A.D. 568, the Northern Zhou Emperor Wudi took a Turk girl, Ashina, as his wife. She brought music and dance from Kucina, Shule and Bokhara and Samarkand (the area of Samarkand in the modern-day Uzbek Soviet Socialist Republic) with her to Chang'an. The artists who came with her to the Central Plains gave music and dance performances which were rich in ethnic colour and aroused great interest. Thus music and dance from the Western Regions began to have a greater influence on the Central Plains. Other kinds of music and dance from places such as India and Korea also entered China during the two Jin and Southern and Northern Dynasties.

"Xiliang Music" which also had quite an influence was introduced to the Central Plains during the Southern and Northern Dynasties. Xiliang is in the area of modern Gansu but was then a gateway for communications between the central areas and the Western Regions. Music and dance from this area had its own unique style, formed from an assimilation of that of the Han and of other nationalities (principally Kucina) in the Western Regions. "Xiliang Music" enjoyed unabated popularity for the several hundred years from the time of the Southern and Northern Dynasties until the Sui and Tang. The introduction of national minority music and dance then paved the way for the flourishing of music and dance during the Sui and Tang dynasties as well as for the establishment of ritual court festival music such as the "Seven Books of Music", "Nine Books of Music" and "Ten Books of Music" (each of these also included dance). The piece "The King of Lanling Goes into Battle" which originated during the Northern Qi (A.D. 550-577) and the "City Dance" created during the Northern Zhou (known in the Tang as Bokhara Music) all continued into the Tang and were further developed.

The "Variety Shows", much in vogue under the Han, still circulated widely during the Southern and Northern Dynasties at folk, court and religious activities in both southern and northern parts of the country. Buddhism was very popular at the time so there were frequent performances of various folk arts at religious festivals. The *Description of Buddhist Temples of Luoyang* written by Yang Xuanzhi who lived at the end of the Northern Wei (A.D. 386-534) and during the Eastern Wei (A.D. 534-550) gives an account of what a splendid sight the shrines and pagodas in the temples at Luoyang had been before the military turmoil. The book also tells of the dissolute life the ruling class led under the cloak of religion and writes about the great spectacle at parades for Buddhist statues from the temples or at performances of song and dance variety shows within the temple compounds. For example, the procession for the Buddha at Changqiu Temple was "led by a lion for driving away evil spirits" (a folk lion dance) as well as acrobatic performances of "sword swallowing and fire spitting". At Jingle Temple "dancing girls were often present, songs filled the air. Dancing sleeves slowly turned ... ushering in all kinds of music and displays of acrobatics within the compound. Strange beasts tumbled and danced in the halls" (this was in fact the Bird and Animal Dance from the Han variety shows). The temples used traditional popular arts for spreading religion and increasing their influence. Through such activities popular arts were preserved and improved on and mass entertainment made use of the opportunity to develop.

With the move southwards of the Han political centre and many of the Han themselves, their traditional music and dance was brought from the north into the region south of the Changjiang (Yangtze). Folk song and dance were also extremely popular there at the time. A description of the strength of dance under the Song Emperor Wendi, (A.D. 424-453) is contained in the section "Biographies of Upright Officials" from the *History of the Southern Dynasties*: "In every populated area, every market town, song and dance proliferate." Or else, take the example of Qianxi Village in the south of Deqing County, Zhejiang. It was an area where performers flocked together with several hundred households studying music there. So many artists came from the place that it gave rise to the expression "Dance comes from Qianxi." Qianxi was also the name for a dance said to have originated under the Jin and popular throughout the Southern Dynasties. As Liu Shan who lived during the Chen Dynasty (A.D. 557-589) writes in the line of a poem "Dancing the Qianxi above the pond". The Qianxi Dance was preserved in the "Music of Qingshang" of the Tang Dynasty. A poet from that period, Cui Hao, writes in a poem "Most cherished is the Qianxi Dance in green costume." In "Climbing the Eastern Tower in Changsha on the Ninth Day to Watch Dances" Li Qunyu, also of the Tang, mentions the "Qianxi" and "Green Waist" dances together. Evidently then, the Qianxi Dance was a refined dance for women.

The ruling class of the Southern Dynasties always laid great store by singing, dancing and music-making. Though living in a period of great unrest they held idle chatter in esteem and believed in making merry whenever they could. Large numbers of dancing girls were kept in their households, the art of song and dance had become a mere object for their pleasure. Court nobles adopted many folk songs and dances. The "Music of Qingshang" in vogue during the Southern Dynasties was in fact traditional songs and dances which had been popular in the Han national area since the dynasty of the same name. From the Eastern Jin on, the "Music of Qingshang" was introduced into the south. Folk music and dance originally there (Western Tunes, Songs of Wu) continued to emerge and enrich its contents. The Emperors Xiaowen and Xuanwu of the Northern Wei conquered the Huaihe and Hanshui river valleys and acquired old compositions from the Central Plains as well as Southern music and dance in circulation there. Following the practice under the Southern Dynasties it continued to be called the Music of Qingshang. Thus this compilation which had been prevalent in the South, was introduced into the North.

In line with developments at the time the contents of the "Music of Qingshang" broadened to include many folk songs and music from both North and South plus dance music and songs to match the dancing performances. For example, the "Bayu Dance", "Scarf Dance", "Bi Dance" (a kind of Drum Dance), "Duo Dance" (a *duo* was like a bell) were included. The selection also contained dances of the Wu Kingdom in the lower Yangtze area during the period of the Three Kingdoms such as the "Whisk Dance", "White Ramie Dance" and the Jin Dynasty "Dance of Mingjun". During the Southern Dynasties some of these dances gradually became ritualized through being used in votive rites at local temples. A few of the pieces in the "Music of Qingshang" were worked on by artistes who polished them into exquisite dances. An example is the "White Ramie Dance" originally a folk dance from the lower Yangtze area. It took its name from the costumes which were made from white ramie. Subsequently it was introduced into court and often danced at banquets, enjoying unbroken popularity for the 500 or 600 years from the Jin up until the Sui and Tang dynasties. Poets under these dynasties wrote much poetry about the "White Ramie Dance". Though some of them spread the mistaken idea prevalent in the upper segments of society that people should make merry whenever they could and sometimes even included lines praising this section of the community, many gave strikingly detailed descriptions of spectacular performances of the "White Ramie Dance". They almost make the reader see the image of a beautiful young woman, dressed in a long-sleeved dancing costume which was "as light as cloud and of a silver hue". Her head sparkled with pearl and jade ornaments. As the music slowly picked up, she sang in a lilting voice. The young woman danced with light, delicate steps as she raised her sleeves which rose and fell like a swan in flight with a slow measured motion. As she stopped for a moment, her flashing eyes swept the audience, she gently moved or rather did not move but seemed propelled forward. Cocking her head, she spun round gently. At times she slowly swept across the long sleeves to brush her face and at others flapped them like billowing snow as her nimble dance steps quickened in tempo. The rich urgent strains of the orchestra, her ethereal, floating dance movements... what a captivating performance! However, concealed behind such beautiful scenes was the terrible suffering of the song and dance artists — mere objects to provide pleasure for others, slaves with no personal freedom who could be thrown out at any time. Life had only humiliation and grinding poverty in store for them. The tragic state of mind of the song and dance artists was mirrored to a certain extent in a few such poems.

Let us now look then at the hard lot of Lü Zhu, a dancing girl famous in the Jin Dynasty. A cruel and greedy bureaucrat landlord called Shi Chong lived at the time. He kept a personal troupe of several hundred song and dance girls. He often ordered them to get his guests to drink. If the guest did not, Shi Chong had the girl killed. He bought Lü Zhu, a well-known dancing girl, with pearls. She was of great beauty and could play the flute. Her rendering of the "Dance of Mingjun" was very famous. It told the tale of "Zhaojun Going Across the Frontier". Zhaojun lived during the Western Han and was picked to enter the court under the reign of the Emperor Yuandi. In 33 B.C., Huhanxie, a Hun chieftain from the Northern frontier, came to the court and proposed marrying into the Western Han as a way of settling disputes — a common practice in those days. Zhaojun herself asked to be married to Huhanxie and followed her husband back amongst the Huns. Her story formed a popular theme for poems, plays and novels thereafter. It is possible that the actions to the "Dance of Mingjun" were tailored to the words of the song. Later on, Prince Sima Lun of Zhao, took over completely. He had differences with Shi Chong so one of his henchmen, Sun Xiu, got some people to ask the landlord for Lü Zhu, on purpose. Shi Chong refused whereupon Sima Lun had him arrested and his house confiscated. On his arrest, Shi Chong said to Lü Zhu, "I have been wronged because of you." Under such pressure Lü Zhu was forced to kill herself by jumping off a building, victim of the power struggle within the ruling class of the Jin Dynasty.

To sum up, the "Music of Qingshang" which was popular during the Southern Dynasties along with "Hu Music" and "Hu Dance" (national minority and foreign music and dance) from the north continued to make their way southwards.

The historical side to this exchange of song and dance between nationalities is fully brought out in representational material of the time. A musician and the figure of a man raising his hand to push back his small hat are portrayed on the neck of a china pot for storing grain (see fig. 40) which dates from the Six Dynasties.* It was unearthed at Rui'an in Zhejiang. Their general attire closely resembles that of national minorities in Xinjiang. Pictures of merry-making and dancing painted in tombs from the Sixteen Kingdoms at Asitana in Turpan, Xinjiang, include one of a girl in a long dress with gathered waist. She glides along dancing with arms stretched straight out to right and left. Such dancing poses appear even now in national minority dances from the area of Xinjiang (see fig. 41). Both the musicians

---

* Name of a period. The states of Wu from the Three Kingdoms and the Eastern Jin and Song, Qi, Liang and Chen from the Southern Dynasties all had their capital at Jiankang (now Nanjing in Jiangsu). Together they are known in history as the Six Dynasties, a general term for the period lasting some 300 years from the beginning of the 3rd century until the end of the 6th century.

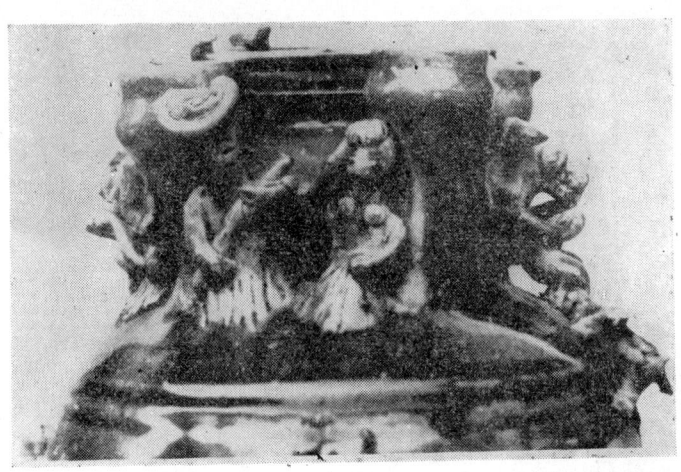

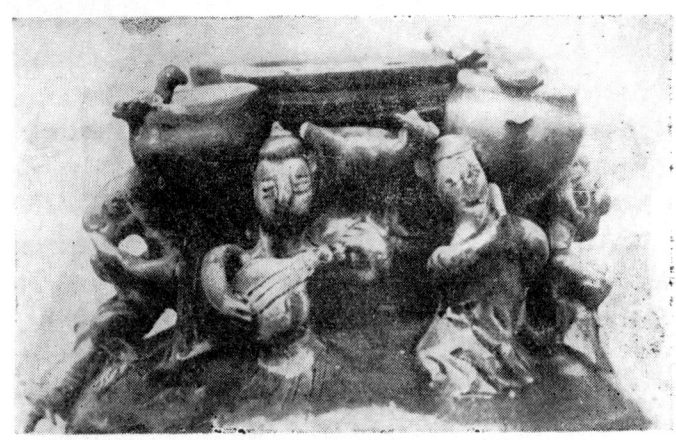

40. A Six Dynasties china pot for storing grain and detail of two figures. Unearthed at Rui'an, Zhejiang.

and dancers in the song and dance picture depicted on the yellow glaze flat porcelain pot unearthed from Fan Cui's tomb of the Northern Qi at Anyang in Henan are figures of "people from the Western Regions" (see fig. 42). On the lotus platform in the centre is a man with his head turned towards the left and his left shoulder slightly raised. His right arm is held up as his feet dance. The accompaniment of four musicians consists of pipes, strings and drums as well as one clapping his hands to the singing. It is a scene full of life. Brick reliefs of the Southern and Northern Dynasties uncovered at Dengxian County in Henan are carved with song and dance scenes strongly characteristic of the Han. One of the dancers is wearing a mask. According to research done by the famous Chinese author and scholar, Shen Congwen, this could possibly be a masked dance called the "Arts of Wenkang" (see fig. 43). The "Annals of Music" in the *History of the Sui Dynasty* says that after the death of Yu Liang of the Jin, his house minstrels created a masked dance in his memory, the "Arts of Wenkang". At the beginning of the Sui, it was included in the "Seven Books of Music". Later, it became the last section of the "Nine Books of Music" — the "End of the Rites". On another of the brick reliefs uncovered at Dengxian County is an engraving of two girls dancing together. Wearing long skirts and large sleeves, they danced with their arms outstretched as they tilt their bodies slightly in a beautiful dancing pose. A figure along-

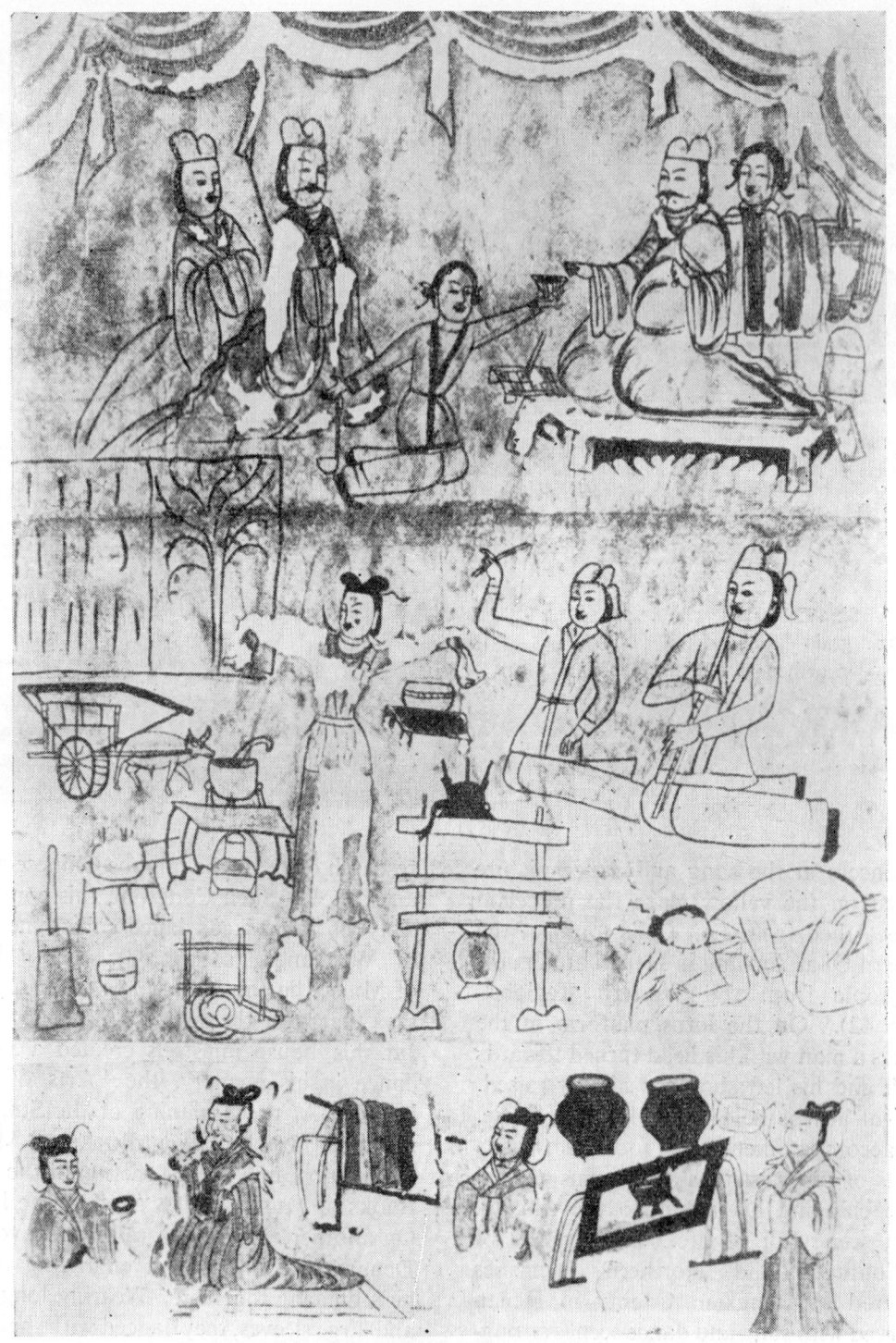
41. Sixteen Kingdoms mural of merry-making and dancing.
Unearthed at Turpan, Xinjiang.

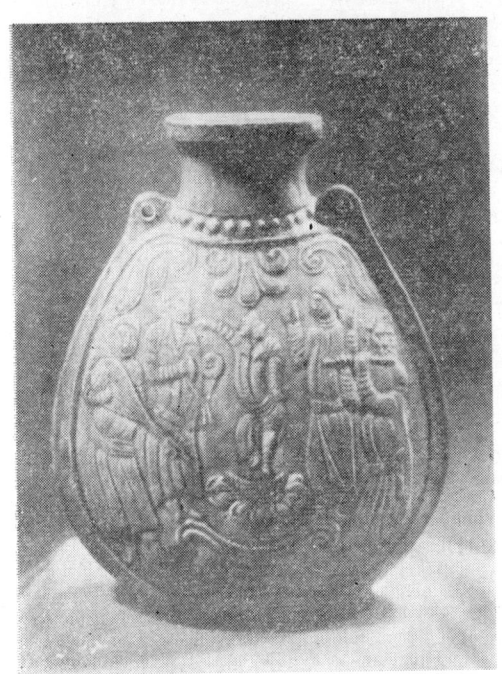 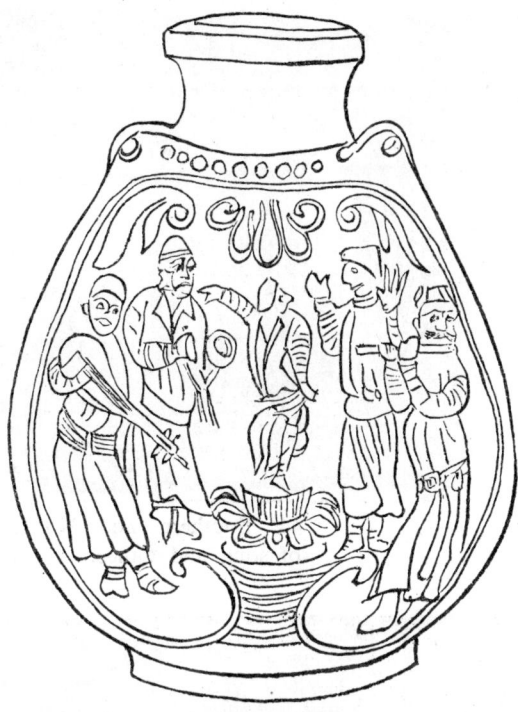

42. Picture of song and dance on a Northern Qi yellow glaze flat pot in porcelain and a copy of its designs. Unearthed at Anyang, Henan.

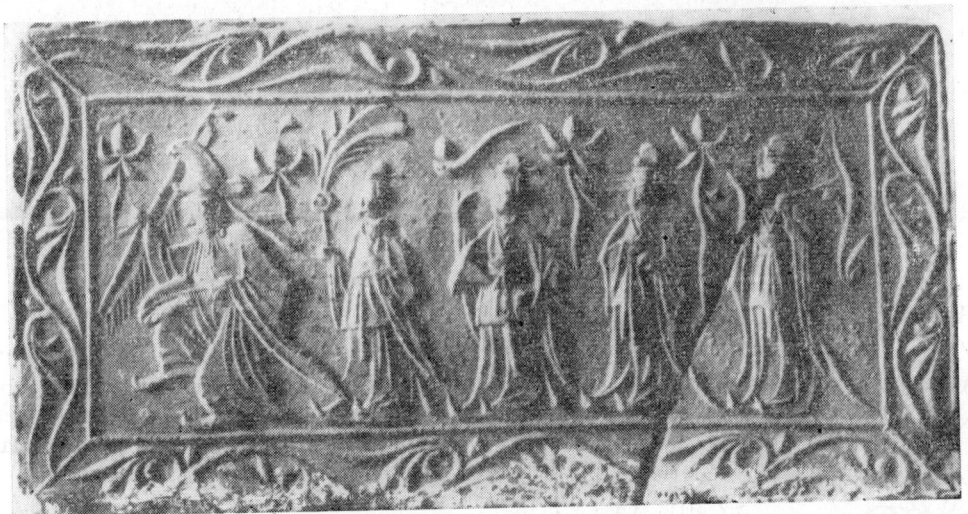

43. Southern and Northern Dynasties brick relief of song and dance. Unearthed at Dengxian, Henan.

side carries a dancing prop made of feathers. Another is beating a waist drum, a third places his hands on his chest (perhaps an accompanying singer) and a fourth is playing a reed-pipe instrument. Both the costumes and dancing poses are in traditional Han style (see fig. 44). Most of these artifacts from coffin chambers portray life as it was

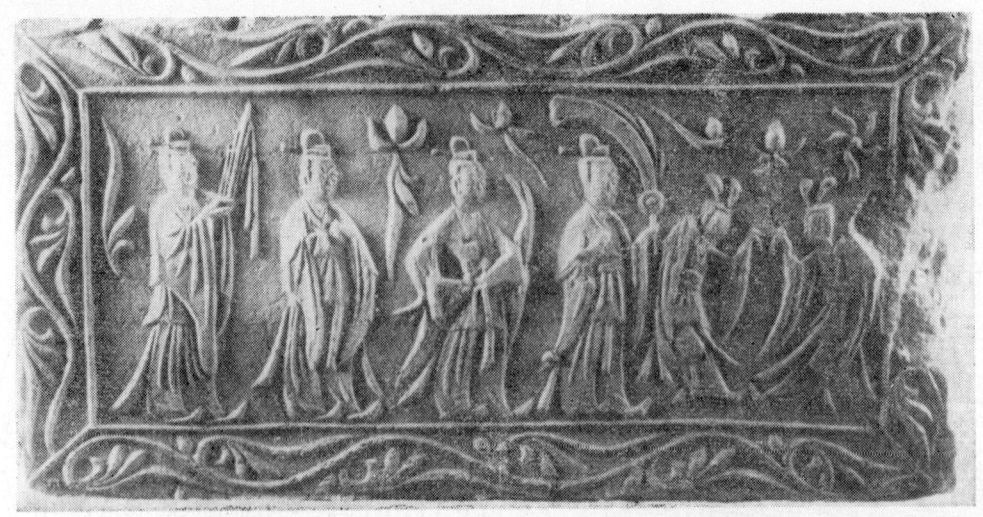

44. Southern and Northern Dynasties brick relief of song and dance. Unearthed at Dengxian, Henan.

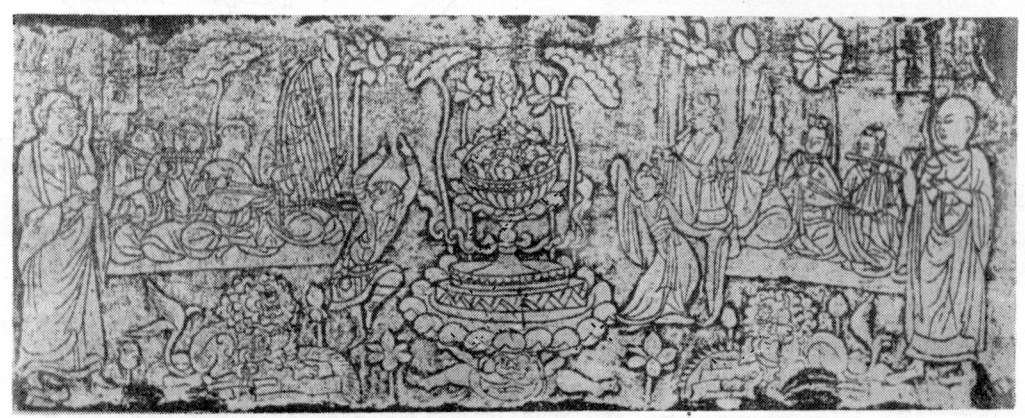

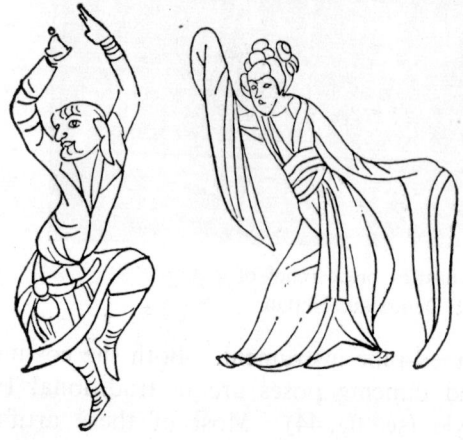

45. Song and dance picture on the ancient plinth for a Buddha from the Southern and Northern Dynasties and copy of a dance detail.

while the dead person was alive. As a result, such figurative work is a fairly faithful reflection of the state of contemporary song and dance.

The incessant upset of war brought great hardship to the population during the Southern and Northern Dynasties. The ruling class made use of religion to lull the minds of the people who because of the terrible suffering put all their hopes in the life to come. Accordingly Buddhism was popular and religious art further developed. A large number of depictions of singers and dancers have been preserved in some of the pictures and carvings which are thus also valuable research materials for studying song and dance then. For example, the murals at Dunhuang in Gansu and the "Heavenly Musicians" of the Northern and Western Wei include string instrument, flute and drum players. Their hand and body postures are strongly reminiscent of the Indian style of dancing. Or like the ancient plinth for a Buddha in Xingping County, Shaanxi (at Huo Qubing's burial ground which survives to this day and has been dated by historians to the time of the Southern and Northern Dynasties) which has a vivid carving of a song and dance scene. In the middle is a large furnace set off by a lotus decoration, to the left a dancing girl dressed in a full-length slim-waisted skirt and broad sleeves (the dress is similar to those of dancing girls on brick reliefs from Dengxian County). Her arms are in a dancing pose similar to "Flag Blowing in the Breeze". To the right of the furnace is a male dancer with a large nose and Western eyes—the figure of a national minority from the Northwest. His clothes are tight fitting and have narrow sleeves. He is holding his arms up high above his head as he stands on tiptoe. Eight accompanying musicians are seated behind (see fig. 45). The fact that a Han was dancing with a member of a national minority who has come to the Central Plains was perhaps the actual situation then!

The two Jin and the Southern and Northern Dynasties were periods of strife but also a time when the culture of different nationalities gradually merged, when various kinds of music and dance arts were exchanged, thus both having an influence on and being absorbed by each other. National and folk song and dance of different styles were widespread in the Central Plains area and greatly enriched the art of Chinese dance thereby preparing the way for the great development in dance during the Tang Dynasty.

CHAPTER SIX
The Tang Dynasty — Golden Age for Dance in Ancient Times

In A.D. 581 the Sui Dynasty unified China and brought to an end the long period torn by war. The Sui carried on and started collecting music and dance from the Southern and Northern Dynasties. This helped the development of music and dance of different nationalities and from different areas as they were better able to copy and absorb things from each other.

To demonstrate the merits of a unified state and the power of the country, the rulers amassed the traditional songs and dances of the Han, of minority nationalities and those which had been introduced from abroad. Early in the reign of the founding Sui Emperor Wendi (581 A.D.-circa 585), the "Seven Books of Music" were drawn up, namely the "Xiliang Arts", "Qingshang Arts", "Korean Arts", "Indian Arts", "Bokhara Arts", "Kucina Arts" and "Arts of Wenkang" (a Han masked dance), seven sections in all. Later on, during the reign of Daye (A.D. 605-616) in the Sui Dynasty another two books, the "Samarkand Music" and "Shule Music" were added to form the "Nine Books of Music". These were all music and dances from previous dynasties which had already been introduced into the Central Plains. They were not just performed in the court then but circulated amongst the population too. An example is "Kucina Music" which enjoyed a great vogue — even the Sui Emperor Wendi did not succeed in banning it. The attire and dancing posture of the Sui figurines of dancing girls in pale yellow glaze (see fig. 46) are not the same as that in the Han Dynasty as parts from other nationalities' dances had already been incorporated.

Apart from assembling large numbers of artistes to strengthen the court music and dance institutions, song, dance and variety shows were brought to the capital to perform every year under the Sui. The main purpose behind this was a definite political one — to flaunt the power and prosperity of the country and the cultural attainments of the Central Plains. Moreover the state of folk song and dance at the time is also apparent from such records as the "Annals of Music" in the *History of the Sui Dynasty*. It relates that in A.D. 606 musicians were brought from all over the country to put on spectacular performances at a reception for some Turk visitors to the capital. Every first lunar month, foreign emissaries flocked to the capital Chang'an (modern Xi'an, Shaanxi). Stages stretched for four kilometres and as many as 30,000 people took part. There were all kinds of acrobatic and magic shows as well as song and dance performed by men in women's roles. In A.D. 601 chieftains of the minority nationalities bearing local specialities as tribute came to the court. Yet again there was a grand display of all types of shows on Tianjin Street. There

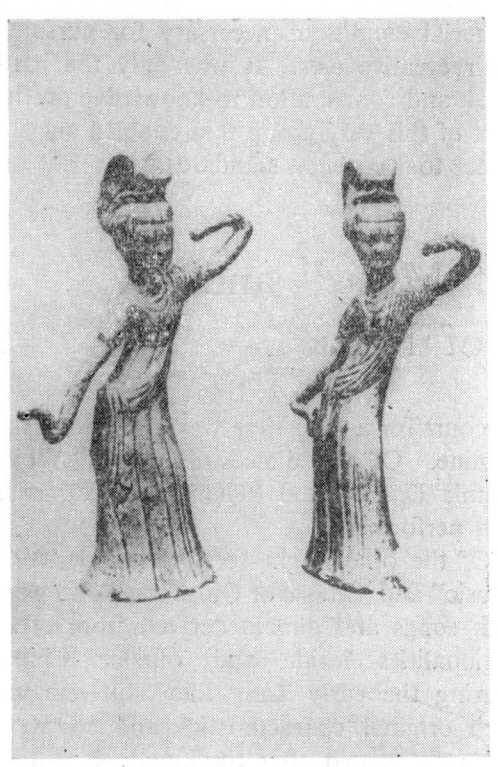

46. Sui figurines of dancing girls in pale yellow glaze.

were up to 18,000 performers, the instrumental music being loud enough to be heard many kilometres away. It really was an exceptionally lavish event.

The Sui poet Xue Daoheng gives a fairly vivid description of mass entertainment at a festival in one of his poems. It was that of the Lantern Festival on the 15th of the first month in the lunar calendar. Crowds of people dressed in their best thronged Chang'an and Luoyang. There were all sorts of performances. Lanterns which were lit all night long hung everywhere. Amidst the rejoicing crowds the sound of singing and music rose and fell. "Qiang flutes play Gansu tunes, Hu dances are performed to Kucina music, masks decorated with gold and silver, festive dress aquiver with pearls and jade." These would have been music and dance performances by national minorities. There were thrilling displays of horsemanship and spell-binding acrobatic and conjuring turns. Also included were many kinds of bird and animal dances: "All the animals dance to and fro, the waddling of the five fowl show, lion cubs with spotted legs, large elephants with their trunks hanging down, goats kneeling and jumping round, riders on white horses wheeling back and forth". Of even greater interest are the equivalent descriptions of scenery in the poem. These "Elephant People" acting the part of animals performed in an area set with scenery very similar to that in the scene from a variety show described in Zhang Heng's *Rhyme-Prose on the Western Capital*.

The Sui Emperor Yangdi spent large amounts of wealth on a life of self-indulgence. The populace were ground down with such unrelenting cruelty they were forced to rise up in resistance in a peasant revolt. The rebellion swept all before it thus ending the Sui Dynasty after little more than 30 years of rule.

With the setting up of the Tang Dynasty in A.D. 618, national power was strong and the political situation remained fairly stable. The economy flourished, trade with other countries expanded and there were frequent cultural contacts. Conditions favourable to the flowering of literature and the arts had been created.

Poetry, music and dance in the Tang reached a peak and was brilliantly successful. It was the golden age for dance in ancient China.

The institutions set up by the Tang court for music and dance — the Jiaofang, Liyuan and Taichangsi* — pooled a large number of noted folk artistes and trained professional performers in a systematic way. They were dispersed all over the country as official players (working at government offices), camp players (serving army officers) and private players (song and dance artistes in noble households). For the most part they all excelled at singing and dancing. In one way, song and dance artistes in the position of slaves suffered much humiliation and depredation. Yet they did acquire the material conditions necessary for pursuing their creative arts. It was only the hard work and contribution to knowledge on the part of this very group that enabled ancient dance to attain new standards.

The "Nine Books of Music" and the "Ten Books of Music"

The Tang carried on the music and dance from the Sui. Those musicians and dancers appointed to the emperor at court were kept on in their posts, the system of music and dance remaining as they were. The "Nine Books of Music" were performed as of old. It was not until the middle of the Zhenguan period (A.D. 637-642) that the "Nine Books of Music" were re-edited as the "Ten Books". Their contents were "Yan Music", "Music of Qingshang", "Xiliang Music", "Indian Music", "Korean Music", "Kucina Music", "Bokhara Music", "Shule Music", "Samarkand Music" and "Qoco Music" (music and dance from the area of present-day Turpan in Xinjiang).

Of the "Ten Books of Music" only "Yan Music" and the "Music of Qingshang" were Han music and dance. "Yan Music", generally referring to the music and dance performed at banquets, was an eulogy. Legend had it that in A.D. 640 "rainbow-coloured clouds appeared and the waters of the Yellow River turned clear".** People thought it was a good omen. Zhang Wenshou, the court musician, subsequently composed the "Song to Rainbow-Coloured Clouds and Clear Water" to pay tribute to the prosperity of the Tang Dynasty. Later it was set to an orchestral accompaniment to form the first of the "Ten Books of Music".

The "Music of Qingshang" continued into the Sui and Tang dynasties but having been at court for a long time was already on the decline. Of the dances only the "White Ramie Dance" and "Qianxi Dance" were still performed.

Of the other eight sections beside "Yan Music" and "Music of Qingshang", all were folk songs and dances derived from other nationalities inside and outside China. During the early Tang they still retained their original characteristics and so were generally named after the kingdom or area they came from. Such pieces with strong local or national flavour enjoyed great popularity on the Central Plains. The "Samarkand Music" was commonly called the "Dervish Dance" as this national minority dance from the Northwest featured whirl-

---

*The Jiaofang was a Tang government office for administering music and dance at the court which concentrated on work such as the teaching, rehearsal and performance of music, singing, dancing and acrobatic acts not included under ceremonial court music. The Liyuan was a body set up under the Tang Emperor Xuanzong for training song and dance artistes. It was located within the Imperial Gardens to the north of Chang'an. The Taichangsi was an institution which just ran protocol, votive rites and ceremonial court music.

**Feudal government officials often pretended that auspicious omens had appeared somewhere or other. This was to curry favour with the emperor by praising his enlightenment. In fact such events did not necessarily occur.

ing movements. These "whirlwind dances" circulated widely then. A vivid description of the dance is contained in the "Whirling Hu Girl" by the celebrated Tang poet Bai Juyi, (A.D. 772-840). The dancer "Raised both arms at the sound of the strings and drums, gyrating in a frenzied dance like flurrying snow. Tirelessly whirling to left and right, thousands of turns which went on for ever". She spun so quickly "A moving chariot wheel seemed unhurried, a tornado slow" and danced with such speed that "How could she know which way she was facing?" Even today, such beautiful spinning movements requiring a high degree of skill can still be seen in folk dances from the areas of Xinjiang in China and Central Asia. Most "Dervish Dances" were performed by women though occasionally by men. Cavern No. 220 at the Mogao Caves in Dunhuang contains the gorgeous music and dance scene "The Physician from the East Changes the Whole of the Earth" which was painted in A.D. 642. Four dancing girls are standing in a line on a small, round mat. Each is in a different posture dancing gracefully in a most life-like way. Two of them are swirling long scarves in the air, the momentum making the fronts of their costumes and ornaments curl up. Throwing out their arms they spin on the spot in quick tempo. The features of one pose lasting a split second from amongst the spinning dance movements have been captured by the artist. It is a strong and evocative image (see fig. 47). Though this is a religious painting, with dancing celestials as its subject, the painter must have resorted to everyday life in his search for models which he then worked on. Thus this painting can be said to depict to a certain extent one of the dance movements from the "Dervish Dance" — the "whirlwind dance" — which was so popular during the Tang.

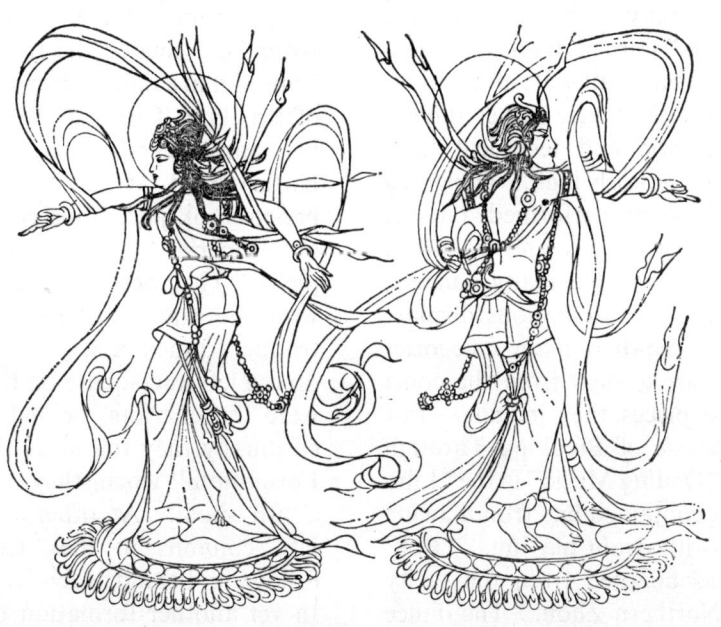

47. Copy of part of the dance on a Dunhuang mural from the early Tang at Cavern No. 220 in the Mogao Caves.

The "Zuobu Arts" and "Libu Arts"

From the mid-Tang on, a lot of minority nationality and foreign music and dance was gradually incorporated into Han music and dance on the Central Plains. A dazzling new form of dance took shape under the Tang.

The overwhelming majority of song and dance pieces in the two main categories of Tang court music and dance — the "Zuobu Arts" and "Libu Arts" — were created during the hundred or more years from the early to the high Tang. Though based on the artistic tradition in the Central Plains, they resulted from incorporating works of minority nationalities and other countries. They were included in the repertoire of song and dance pieces that had been popular for a long time during the Tang. The pieces were no longer named after a country or region but after the name of the score. Each piece of music had a dance to go with it. They were all eulogistic in tone but had nevertheless taken in many folk dance forms.

The "Zuobu Arts" were performed in halls. Characterized by their small scale and limited number of dancers, they were rather refined in style. The artistic and technical level of the performers was fairly high. Generally the "Libu Arts" were performed outside (probably in the courtyards and squares). Large in scale they featured many dancers, the emphasis being on ostentatious display.

The origins of the two main categories described above are evident from the court music and dance pieces they include. For example, the "Music of Breaking Through the Ranks" and "Dading Music" in the "Libu Collection" both contained bits from Kucina music mixed in with drum playing. "Bokhara Music" was adapted from the "City Dance" of the Northern Zhou. The dance had "performers who looked like Qiang Hu people" in it so obviously it was music and dance in the style of a national minority from the north. "Qingshan Music" from the "Zuobu Arts" was styled on the Xiliang area; the "Music of Singing Birds" carried on the tradition of the ancient bird dances and of the "Mynah Dance" from the Jin Dynasty. Wearing mynah bird crests, the performers enacted the dance as birds. All of these pieces praised the ruling emperor yet the form of the dance was derived from the people.

The "Music of Breaking Through the Ranks" was the most famous item in both the Zuobu and Libu Arts. It is said to have been taken to Japan and so was famous abroad as well as in China.

It was a dance adaptation of the "Melody to the Prince of Qin Breaking Through the Ranks", a song in praise of the military exploits of the Tang emperor Li Shimin in unifying the country. Before becoming emperor, Li Shimin had been given the title of the Prince of Qin, hence the piece's title. After he ascended the throne (in A.D. 633) he used it in a dance arrangement, the "Music of Breaking Through the Ranks", based on his many years' experience of life at the battle front. One hundred and twenty people took part (thus easily surpassing the old Imperial "Dance with Sixty-Four People"). They were dressed in armour adorned with silver and carried spears. The dance troupe formed a group which was curved on the left and square on the right. In front were the chariots, behind the troops. Occasionally they fell in as the "Fish in Pairs Formation" when they moved along like a fish shoal. At other times they formed into columns in the "Crane Formation" following behind each other like cranes. In yet another formation the centre opened out like a winnowing fan with both flanks stretched out. The troupe contracted or expanded crisscrossing over until finally the head and tail met up. The dance was divided into three main parts, each had four variations of battle array. There was a large drum as accompaniment, the melody being Kucina Music. Its fast and slow stabbing movements matched the magnificent singing. It was an impressive work with a strong martial air. Although the contents praised the military exploits of the ruler, the feat of arms of Li Shimin did play a definite role in unifying the country so was in keeping with the interests of the people. This was why his praises were sung as well as being the main reason for the dance's great impact and influence both inside and outside of China.

The "Music of Breaking Through the Ranks" was included in the "Libu Arts" during the reign of the Tang Emperor Xuanzong (A.D. 712-756) but still retained its original characteristics as a dance which "spread the martial spirit, and was bellicose in tone". However, the version in the "Zuobu Arts" was a small-scale dance performed by four people. They wore gorgeous red damask silk robes and trousers. It is possible the manner of dancing differed somewhat from that in the Libu Arts. The Emperor Xuanzong had several hundred girls from the court perform it. They are supposed to have danced it quite well — even better than dancers of Taichangsi who often performed it. Probably it was put on for entertainment.

"Taiping Music" from the "Libu Arts" was also known as the "Lion Dance of the Five Directions". Even before the Tang, lion dances circulated amongst the populace. Lions were not native to China. According to the *History of the Late Han Dynasty*, emissaries sent from Indoscythe (now in the area of northeast Afghanistan) and the Kingdom of Arsaces (ancient Persia) brought lions as presents to the Han court. The king of the animals — the lion — was regarded as a symbol of power and fortune. Little by little a form of dance grew out of imitations of the lion's appearance and movements. The "Gazette on Ritual Music" in the *History of the Han Dynasty* mentions "Elephant People" and Yu Kang from the Kingdom of Wei in the Three Kingdoms period says in a note, "Now there are fish, shrimp and lion acts." Clearly then the Lion Dance at the very latest existed by that time. The Lion Dance was also commonly popular during the Southern and Northern Dynasties. The *Description of Buddhist Temples of Luoyang* carries an entry which says that a parade for a statue of the Buddha from Changqiu Temple was "led by a lion for driving away evil spirits. There was sword-swallowing and fire-eating, much leaping around, coloured streamers hung from ropes, peculiar tricks, strange acts and weird clothing. It was the best performance in the capital". At religious festivals, the "Lion Dance" cleared the way ahead. Street corner performances of pole climbing, tight rope walking and acrobatics attracted spectators. By Tang times there had been fairly large improvements and innovations in the "Lion Dance". The "Taiping Music" in the "Libu Arts" was performed on quite a large scale. False lion skins of hair stitched together were worn. Five lions decked out in different colours each stood on their own and portrayed the various moods of the lion such as "crouching, throwing back its head and being friendly". Two other people led the lions by ropes and carried whisks with which to tease them. At the side were some 140 people in a huge accompaniment who sang the song to the "Taiping Dance" out loud. Lions dancing amid this welter of voices must have been quite impressive. Such was the palace "Lion Dance" at the height of the Tang.

When the *Miscellaneous Records from the Board of Music* was written down at the end of the Tang, the "Lion Dance of the

Five Directions" was included under the Kucina Section. The main reason was that the accompaniment, "Taiping Music", was in the same musical style. The dance performance differed from that in the "Libu Arts". There were five lions over three metres tall all in different colours. Each of them had 12 "lion lads" — the people who teased the lion — who wore red headscarves and coloured costumes and carried red whisks. The accompaniment remained the same, "Taiping Music".

A fairly vivid and realistic description of the lion dance is included in Bai Juyi's poem "Xiliang Arts", "In Xiliang Arts a masked Hu plays the lion, head carved in wood, tail of silk, eyes gilded with gold, teeth plated with silver, shaking his costume of hair, waggling both ears". This is almost exactly the same as the "Lion Dance" still common among the people today.

Part of the Song Dynasty *Picture of Children Playing in Spring* shows two children, one behind the other. They are wearing false lion skins. The small face of the child in front is half visible from the mouth of the lion. The child at the back is bent over hidden inside the lion skin, only his legs can be seen. A child in front of the lion looks back as he leads it along by the rope he is carrying. There are three more children at the side with bells and toys. They look as if they are just about to tease the lion. It is an amusing and lively picture of children performing a lion dance (see fig. 48).

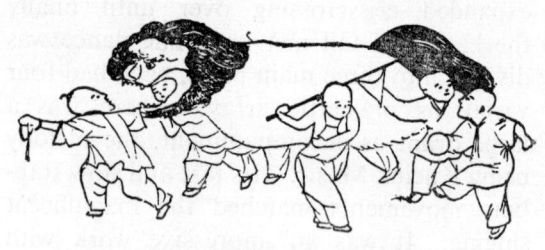

48. Copy of children performing the "Lion Dance" in the Song *Picture of Children Playing in Spring.*

The lion dance in the Qing (1644-1911) painting *A Religious Festival in Beijing* is full of life. There are four lions: a large one in the middle of the picture played by two people; a small lion crouching on the ground at the right which is acted by a single person; another two "small lions" on the left hand side, each played by just one person. They look as if they are playing together. Another two people carrying "whisks" made from tied cloth make "bow and arrow steps" as they tease the lion (see fig. 49). As well as being identical to the description in the Tang poem, this scene is also very similar to both folk and stage performances of the "Lion Dance" today. Clearly although there have been developments and changes during the 1,000 years or more for which the Lion Dance has been circulating, it has all along retained those traditional performing conventions which are intrinsic to it. It is a folk dance steeped in history.

Jian and Ruan Dances

The small-scale dances often performed at ordinary banquets or on other occasions during the Tang were divided into two main categories: "Jian (Energetic) Dances" and "Ruan (Soft) Dances". Jian Dances called for robust agility whereas the Ruan Dances were mostly rather beautiful and sedate.

Of the Jian Dance types, the "Sabre", "Mulberry Branch", "Dervish" (previously explained in the "Samarkand Music" in the "Ten Books of Dances") and "Tartar Prancing" were quite famous.

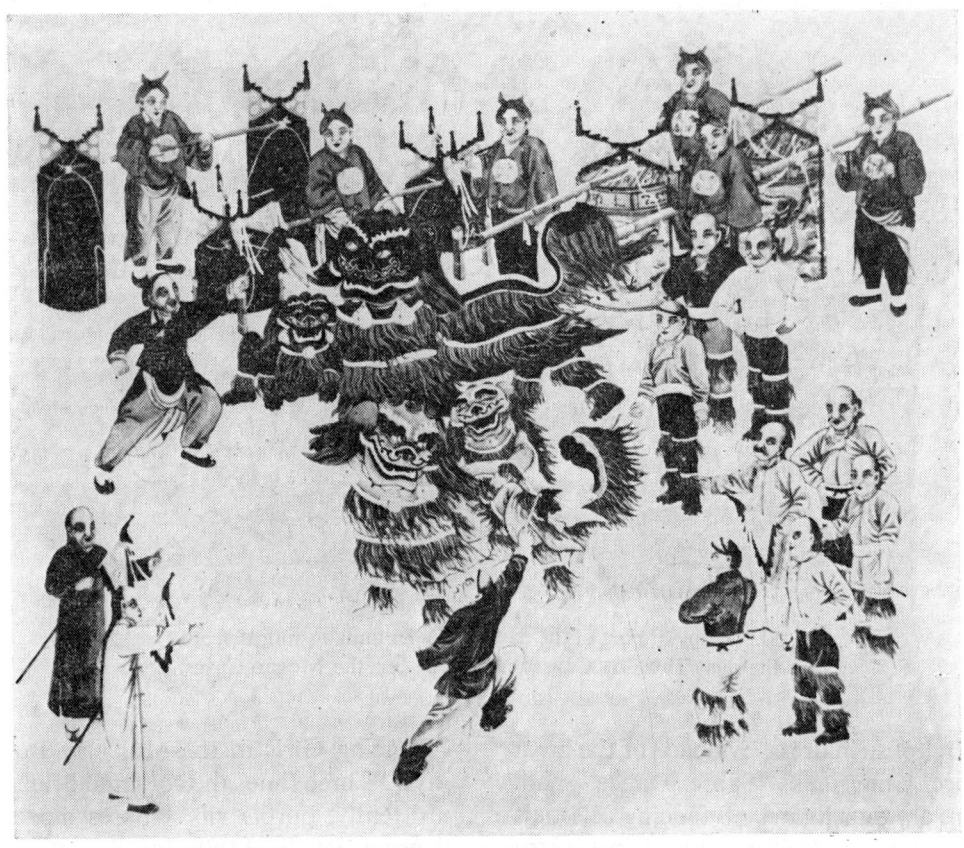

49. "Lion Dance" in the Qing painting *A Religious Festival in Beijing*.

The "Sabre Dance" probably developed from sword play in popular martial arts. A sabre was carried during the dance. The most accomplished exponent of the dance was the celebrated Tang dancer Gongsun. In his poem "Watching a Pupil of Gongsun in the Sabre Dance"; the great Tang poet Du Fu (A.D. 712-770) says he saw Li Shi'er, a pupil of Gongsun, perform it at Kui in A.D. 767. He was overcome by his feelings as he recalled the moving scene 52 years earlier, that is in A.D. 715, when as a child he saw Gongsun herself in the same dance and wrote this poem.

The poem describes how Gongsun's "Sabre Dance" was famous far and wide. People used to flock to see it. As she began to dance light spread in all directions like when Houyi shot down the nine suns*. Her strong, flowing movements resembled the hovering of a dragon bearing the Immortals. In time to the drums' heavy beat there would be a sudden switch to a wild, continuous dance movement, the calm studied movements scattered like light on the waves of a great river. A smart military uniform which had been artistically embellished was worn in the "Sabre Dance" so it had a martial yet decorative air. Du Fu says Gongsun had "a face of jade, clothes of silk". Girls then were

---

*Houyi was the chief of a barbarian tribe from the East during the Xia Dynasty. He was an excellent archer. A Chinese legend says that during the reign of Yao, ten suns rose together. Plants shrivelled up and beasts of prey and snakes wrought havoc. Houyi shot down nine of the suns and killed the beasts and snakes thus alleviating the people from this scourge.

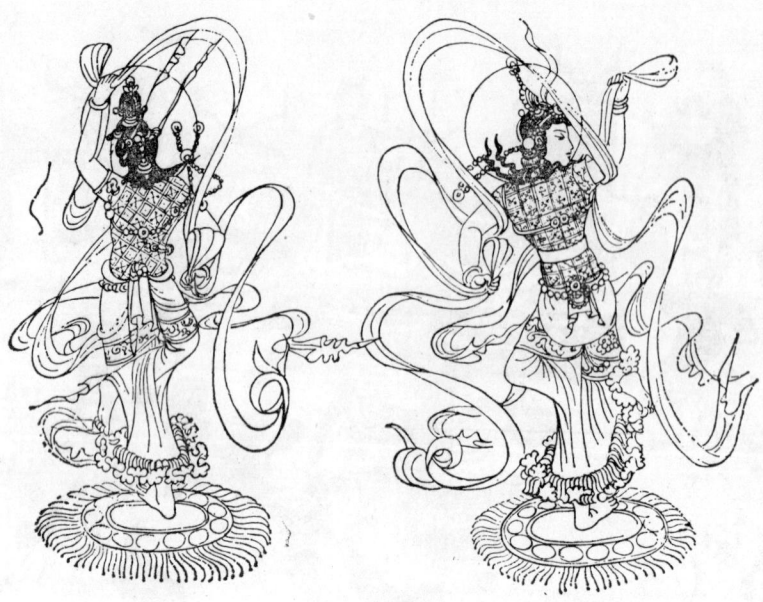

50. Copy of part of the dance on a Dunhuang mural from the early Tang at Cavern No. 220 in the Mogao Caves.

very fond of such dress, evidence of the great influence Gongsun's "Sabre Dance" had.

There are four figures of dancing celestials painted on an early Tang mural in Cavern No. 220 at the Mogao Caves in Dunhuang. Two of them wear conical crowns, "cotton half-sleeves" and "pomegranate skirts". The style and pattern of the dress is reminiscent of a suit of armour, very like a glamourized uniform. The dancing postures are bold and vigorous as if they are straining to stretch upwards (see fig. 50). Could it not contain traces from the "Sabre Dance"?

The "Mulberry Branch Dance" was a folk dance brought from Central Asia. With drums as the main accompaniment it had a clear, strong rhythm. The dancers had to be slim and needed considerable grounding in their art before they could perform it. Zhang Xiaobiao, a Tang poet, writes in the poem "Mulberry Branches", "At their entrance the dancers in the Mulberry Branches are greeted by drumming; fine coloured silk blouses, slim waists." Bai Juyi in "Dancing Girls in the Mulberry Branches" says, "Three times the coloured drum sounds insistently, purple silk blouses move as the dancers int he Mulberry Branches enter." Both poems describe the dancers as they come out on stage to the sound of drumming. There were a large number of variations in the choreography including both vigorous and graceful movements. The long sleeves of the dancers rose up in response to the beat of the drum or hung down to touch the ornate carpet. They danced to the swift, complex rhythm in brocade boots as the gold bells on their headdresses tinkled sweetly. The audience marvelled at the grace of the movements. "Bodies as light as if they had no bones; the onlookers were amazed," (from a poem by Liu Yuxi). As the performance drew to a close, the dancers made a low bending movement, their blouses soaked through with perspiration. "The drums' fierce beat urges on limp bodies; sweat drenched silk costumes, flowers spattered with rain" (poem by Liu Yuxi). With the dance's wide circulation, "Mulberry Branch Dancers" emerged to perform the work so it obviously required special skill and ability. Although originally a solo dance, a "Double Mulberry Branch" version performed by two people appeared later. According to an introduction to a "Poem to the Mulberry Branches" from the Board of Music it was "Danced by two girls, their headdresses decorated with gold bells. On a tapping roll from the drums they come on stage hidden in two lotuses. They appear when the petals split open. The girls dance together in a performance which incorporates elegance and refinement." The two girls first hid in lotus flowers then as the petals slowly opened came out to dance. What a picturesque form it took. A broken Tang stone tablet in Shaanxi Provincial Museum has a lion and creeper pattern carved on either side. The middle part of the design shows two people dancing dressed in long-sleeved dance costumes. They wear hats decked with floating streamers. Each steps with one foot on the lotus flower, bending the other leg in front as they dance in harmony together sweeping up their sleeves (see fig. 51). Could this be the "Double Mulberry Tree" in which they have first been concealed inside the lotus emerging to dance after it has opened? Of even greater interest are the features of the dancers on either side of the stone tablet for they are quite different. On one side is a clear-featured Han, on the other a large nosed "person from the Western Regions" with deep-set eyes. The dancing pose is however identical. It attests to the fact that the Han used to dance this piece with people from the Western Regions.

The "Tartar Prancing Dance" was brought from Chaj (the area of modern Tashkent in the Uzbek Soviet Socialist Republic). Most of the performers were "people from the Western Regions" whose "skin was like jade and noses like owls". They wore conical hats and "Hu robe" with narrow

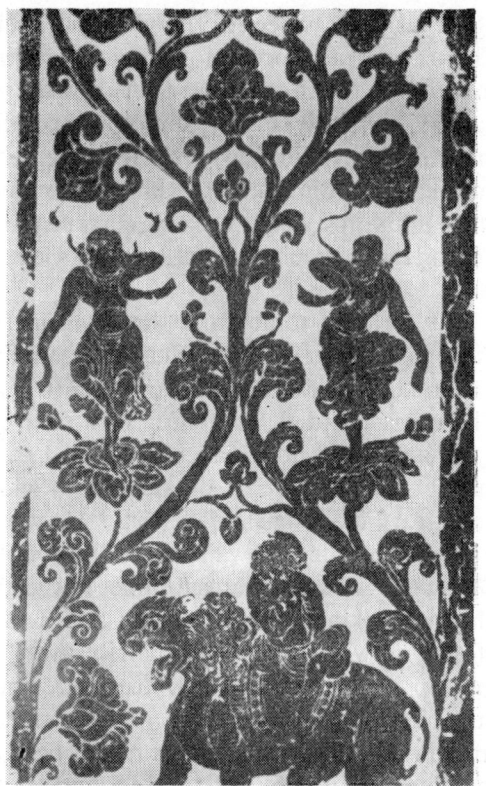

51. Rubbing from one side of the broken Tang tablet of lions, creeper patterns and pictures of people dancing.

sleeves. They rolled up the fronts and backs of the robe to make it easier when dancing. A long belt with grape designs was tied at their waists and hung down one side. Their soft boots were of a beautiful brocade. They performed on a carpet. At the start, the dancers sometimes gulped down a glass of wine, throwing it down before beginning to dance. At other times they first said a few words in their own tongue and then danced once again. Probably the manner of dancing varied somewhat according to differences in the occasion of the performance and audience. The "Tartar Prancing Dance" consisted mainly of leaps and a swift tramping step which changed frequently. Following the rapid tempo of the music, they danced the same step again and again as they wheeled round in a circle. There were all sorts of variations during the dance which was performed with panache. Similarly highly skilled dances for men which include many leaping movements and have a complicated rhythm for the dance steps and a lusty style are still current today among those circulating in the area of Central Asia.

The Su Sixu tomb from the Tang in the Eastern suburbs of Xi'an, Shaanxi, contains a mural of musicians and dancers (see fig. 52). There is a bearded Hu dancer with deep-set eyes and high nose dancing on a carpet in the middle. He is dressed in a white head scarf and long-sleeved shirt. He wears a black belt round his waist and yellow boots. On either side are ranged nine musicians playing all kinds of instruments and a pair of singers who are singing merrily away at the top of their voices with arms stretched out. The left leg of the dancer stands straight while the right one is raised bent at the knee. His left arm is held up above his head, the right arm hangs down. He is looking down as if in a dancing pose where he has just landed back on the ground after leaping into the air. The dancer is a male "Hu". His attire and dance posture bear similarities to the "Tartar Prancing Dance" described in Tang poems. Though it is difficult to determine whether this is in fact the "Tartar Prancing Dance" so popular in the Tang Dynasty, it does at the very least provide valuable reference material for studying the subject.

The "Green Waist Dance" was the most famous of the "Ruan Dances". A story goes that during the Zhenyuan years (A.D. 785-804) of the Tang, a musician presented a piece of music to the Emperor Dezong. The emperor ordered him to make extracts of the most important or beautiful passages in the work which then went to form the "Green Waist". An extremely popular tune of the time, it was firmly rooted in folk music. Possibly the musician had made his own arrangement of a popular song as many of the court musicians then were accomplished folk artists. The "Green Waist" from the "Ruan Dances" was a solo dance for women set to the same music.

Li Qunyu, a Tang poet, wrote, "The women from the South are beautiful, in the graceful Green Waist Dance.... They gilde like emerald orchids, graceful as swimming

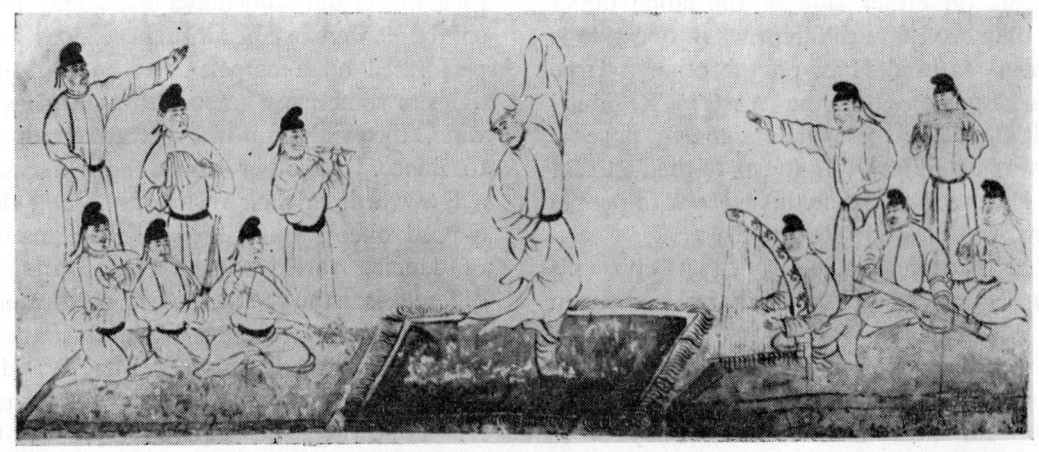

52. Tang mural of musicians and dancer. Unearthed at Xi'an, Shaanxi.

dragons.... Their slow deportment seems never-ending, as with complex gestures the piece nears its end. Bending and turning like lotuses breaking the waves, flurrying as scattered snow in the wind. Lowering their heads they give lingering looks, long robes sweeping into the air. Worried only that they cannot be caught, but will fly off following startled geese." The beautiful choreography at a performance of this dance is movingly described.

The Southern Tang (A.D. 937-975) in the Five Dynasties period inherited parts of the creative legacy from the Tang. The painting *At Han Xizai's Evening Party* shows Wang Wushan in the "Green Waist Dance" (see fig. 53). She is wearing a narrow-sleeved sky blue dancing costume with a long front. Though her back is to the audience, her face is partially visible over her right shoulder. The right foot is slightly raised ready to be brought down. Both hands are behind her back just about to be pushed down and out to sweep up her long sleeves. Such clear evidence about period, circumstances, dancer and dance piece is extremely rare in figurative materials on ancient dance. Only one drum and a pair of clappers are being used in a very simple accompaniment. Clearly then the scene shown is of an impromptu performance. However, the very fact that this old painting exists means that even 1,000 years later we can still see a pose from the "Green Waist Dance".

The "Green Waist Dance" was included among the "Ruan Dances" in the Jiaofang of the Tang Dynasty. There were even people performing it down in the South far away from the capital. Han musicians in the Tang Dynasty also took the music to the Tibetan Plateau when they played it at a banquet given by the king in honour of a court emissary. Clearly the piece was widely popular.

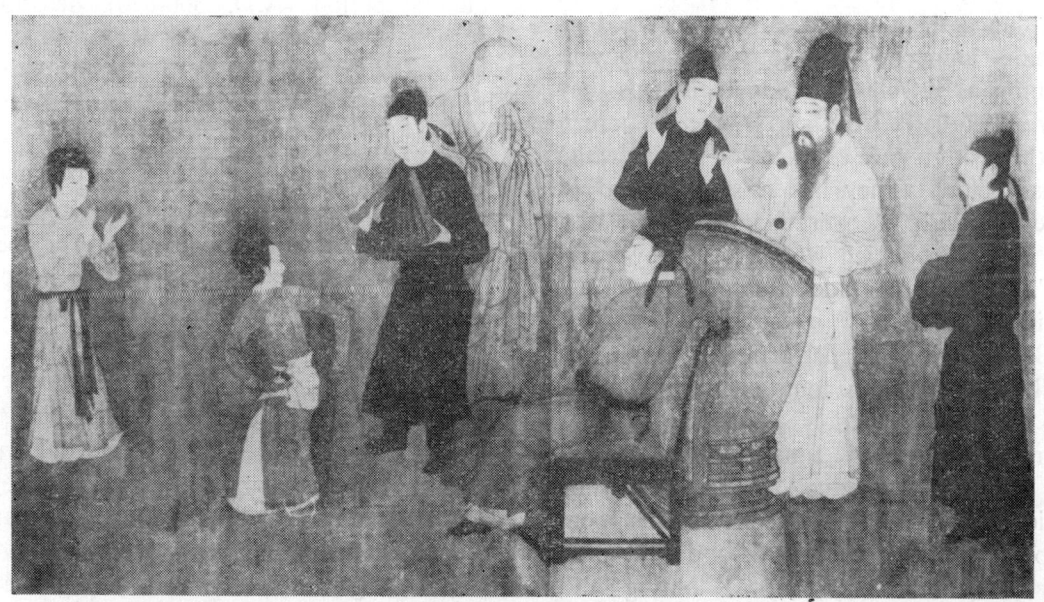

53. Wang Wushan dancing the "Green Waist Dance" in the painting *At Han Xizai's Evening Party* from the Southern Tang in the Five Dynasties period (section).

Grand Song and Dance Compositions

These "Grand Compositions" were composite song and dance pieces comprising music, dancing and poetry. To begin with there was an instrumental passage called the "Free Introduction" which had no fixed tempo. Next came a song in slow time (sometimes dance was included as well) the "Middle Introduction". Finally the rhythm quickened for a dance piece, the "Finale", with its rising and falling variations.

"Rainbow-Coloured and Feathered Costumes" was a grand song and dance composition famous in Tang times. The score was said to have been a partial adaptation of Indian "Brahman music" by the Tang Emperor Xuanzong with the dance being set to it. It was often performed at banquets at court and for high nobles. The most famous performance was that of Yang Yuhuan, Xuanzong's favourite concubine. For the dance the performers were dressed as female immortals in clothes which were glamorous yet elegant. On their tops they wore "Feathered Costumes"— peacock green clothes with a pale coloured or silvery white dress below. They had a special kind of ceremonial shawl over their shoulders and a "headdress which wobbled as they walked". Pearls and jade ornaments adorned their bodies.

Before the dance performance began, the orchestra played a long melodious piece, the "Free Introduction" consisting of solos or rounds with no set time. There followed the "Middle Introduction" in slow time which brought out the dancers. In his poem "Song of Rainbow-Coloured and Feathered Costumes" Bai Juyi says 'Floating and wheeling, light as swirling snow; moving coyly sideways like a swimming dragon. Her hands behind her, she is as limp as a willow. When she trails the front of her gown, cloud seems to emerge." These vivid lines metaphorically describe the delicate pirouettes, smooth flow of dance steps, graceful dancing movements and ethereal quality of the dance. After the "Finale", the rhythm quickened. Rapid dance actions made the waist ornaments and hat tassles jump to and fro. The dancing suddenly stopped after a swift burst of rhythm and the entire work ended with a slow passage of music which "held one note".

The form of the dance performance was not entirely fixed. Versions of "Rainbow-Coloured and Feathered Costumes" performed at some periods of the Tang court differed. In A.D. 745 when Yang Yuhuan was made a high-ranking courtesan and thereafter, all her performances of this dance at the Lily Magnolia Palace were solos. The one Bai Juyi saw at the palace during the Yuanhe period (A.D. 806-820), described in the poem was a pas de deux. In it he writes, "At the Lantern Festival nodding head greets the green buds, the Heavenly Queen parts from the young girl with a toss of the sleeve," a description of two dancers changing place as they drew close together or separated flicking their sleeves. The poem finally says that he had taught two people, Li Juan and Zhang Tai, the dance — further evidence that it was a dance for two. In A.D. 836 at the beginning of the Kaicheng period under the Emperor Wenzong, 300 young dancers less than 15 years old were used in a performance of the "Rainbow-Coloured and Feathered Costumes". Later under the Emperor Xuanzong (A.D. 847-859) a large troupe made up of several hundred girls from the palace performed the dance. Dressed in feather costumes with pearl and jade ornaments they carried streamers as they danced gracefully like soaring birds. These large-scale group dances at court were often for effect, though such serried formations were no match in artistic skill for the solo dances or pas de deux.

"Rainbow-Coloured and Feathered Costumes" had definite artistic originality but men of letters were particularly fulsome in their praise of the dance as the emperor had arranged it. This does also mean that a fairly large body of literary material has been left so even today we can still ascertain roughly how it was danced then.

Folk Song and Dance Drama

Many of the dances in the Tang expressed certain feelings in a set style. There were also some which combined singing, dancing and acting in song and dance dramas which portrayed set characters and plot. "Damian", "Botou" and the "Battered Wife" are three examples of the genre famous in the Tang.

"Damian" was a marked dance which originated in the Northern Qi and was very popular during the Tang Dynasty. According to legend Gao Changgong, the Prince of Lanling in Northern Qi, was a brave warrior and very good-looking. He resented not looking more war-like so wore a mask to battle. "The Prince of Lanling Goes into Battle" was written in his honour. The music was later used to create a dance which showed him leading and fighting in battle. When this piece was performed in the Tang, the dancer wore purple costume with a golden belt and carried a whip (i.e. drumstick). It probably represented marching to the sound of drums.

"Botou" is said to have been brought from the Western Regions. Someone living there was eaten by a tiger. His son climbed a mountain to find his father's corpse and kill the tiger. There were eight bends in the mountain and the same number of sections in the piece. The dancer wore mourning clothes. His hair was dishevelled and he looked as if he had been crying.

Both of the above pieces had just one character with a fairly simple plot. They cannot yet be termed full-fledged song and dance dramas. However the "Battered Wife" was fairly complete. A very ugly man called Su was said to have lived at the end of the Song (or during the Northern Qi). He was a heavy drinker and used to return home drunk to beat his wife. She was very beautiful and could sing. She would go in tears to complain to the neighbours following such unprovoked attacks. Gradually a kind of song and dance drama grew out of people's imitations of the sound of her sobbing and the way she was beaten. For the performance a man dressed up as a woman sang and danced. He would shake his body in time to the singing and then when a section had finished, people in the wings would sing in response, "Battered wife, sing back! Battered wife sing back about your troubles." The husband would then come on stage and make beating actions. Probably this section of the performance was rather comical with the image of the ugly husband being played up so they could make the audience laugh. Later on the part of the wife was played by a woman.

A poem by Chang Feiyue of the Tang describes the scene at a performance of this song and dance piece held in a common square. It says that many people clustered round to look as the performers pirouetted round the "stage"—a coloured mat set on the ground. They would raise their arms and tidy their clothes and the crowd would sing back together in chorus. These were powerful spoken parts too. The poet exclaims "How much pity can their hearts take?" Clearly it was quite a moving performance. The piece was a fairly rounded song and dance drama which can be said to be the precursor of later traditional opera.

Music and dance were the main forms of performing art under the Tang. Thanks to accounts in prose and poetry a wealth of written data has been preserved and the murals in caves as well as dancing figurines and pictures uncovered in tombs have also provided us with valuable figurative material. The latter are particularly close to life so all the more realistic and reliable. Since the feudal lords then all kept large numbers of skilled song and dance performers in their houses, dance figurines and murals from the tombs are very probably scenes of song and dance enjoyed by the deceased while alive. The richness and variety of Tang dance is

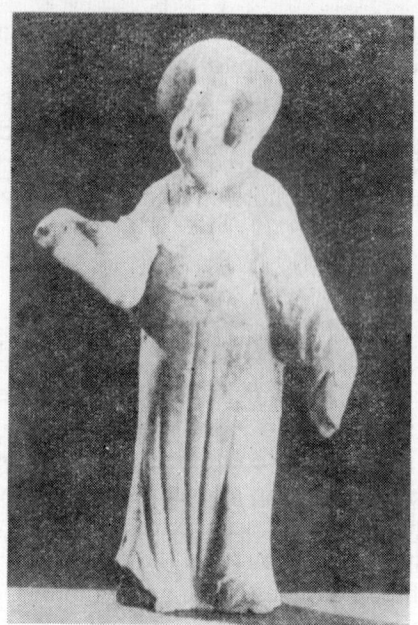

55. Tang figurine of a dancing girl. Unearthed at Xianyang, Shaanxi.

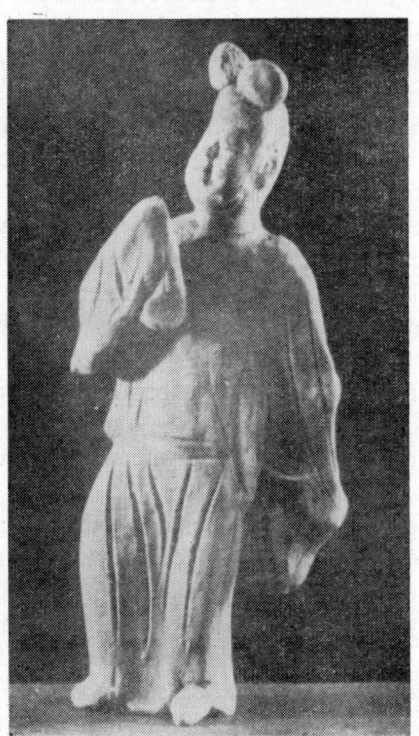

54. Tang figurine of a dancing girl. Unearthed at Xi'an, Shaanxi.

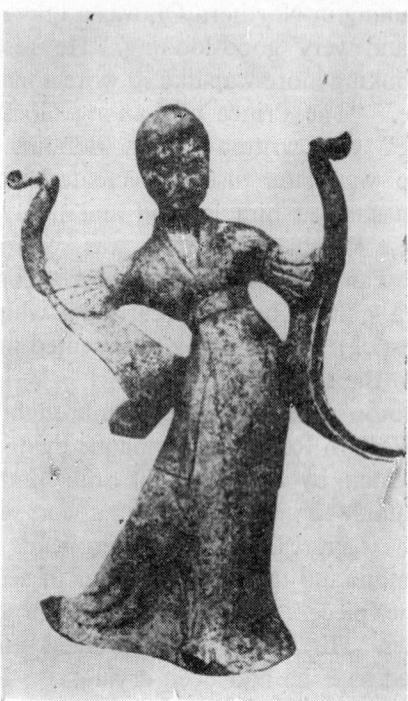

56. Tang figurine of a dancing girl.

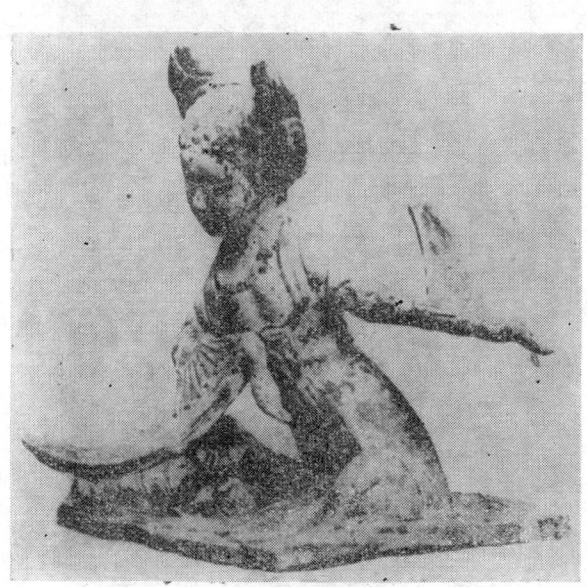

57. Tang painted figurine of a dancing girl.

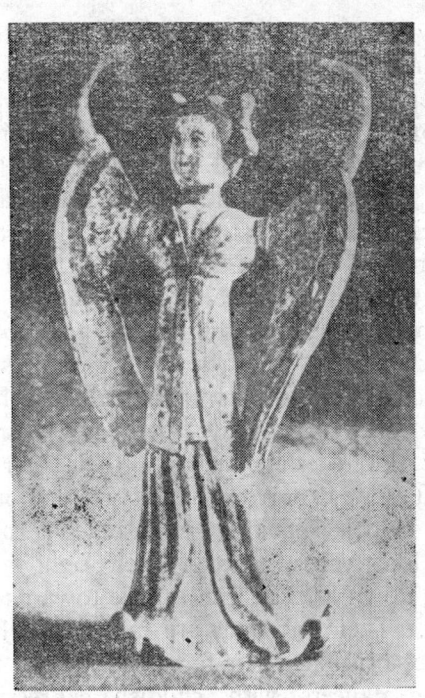

58. Tang figurine of a dancing girl.

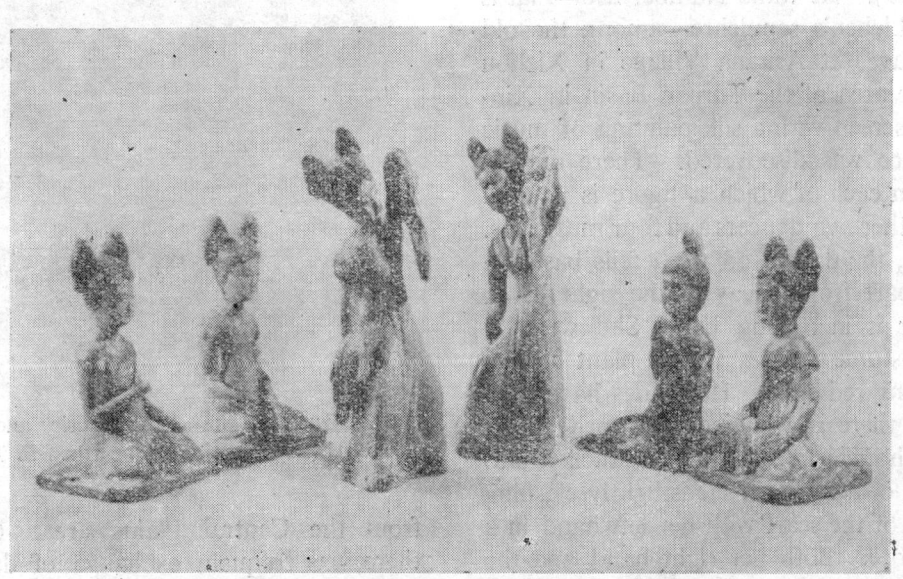

59. Tang painted pottery figures of musicians and dancers. Unearthed at Liquan, Shaanxi.

fully brought out in the particularities of style of each figurine's dress and dance pose which are all quite distinct. Take for example the dance figurines unearthed from Tang tombs in Shaanxi — one at Chayang Village in Xi'an and the other at Dizhangwan in Xianyang. They both wear long-sleeved dancing costumes in the style of robes.

— 63 —

They have tender expressions and seem to be singing as they dance (see figs. 54 and 55). Other Tang dance figurines wear slim-waisted long skirts. Their costumes have narrow sleeves which widen at the cuff. They look very beautiful as they wave their arms dancing (see figs. 56, 57 and 58). The tomb of Zheng Rentai in Liquan County, Shaanxi was one of the accompanying tombs near Zhaoling, the tomb of the Tang Emperor Taizong. The painted pottery figures of musicians and dancers unearthed there have been portrayed in a lively way. A pair of clear skinned dancing girls, their hair up in buns, wear narrow-sleeved white blouses with short jackets in red as an outer garment and long yellow skirts. Their right arms hang down as they lean a little towards the right. Their left arms are raised, the long sleeves brushing their faces. They are two young dancers with childish expressions (see fig. 59). At tomb Number 230—that is Zhang Lichen's sepulchre—among the old Tang graves at Asitana Village in Xizhou (now the area of the Turpan Basin in Xinjiang) a screen with a silk painting of music and dance was discovered. There are six panels on each of which a figure is painted —altogether two dancers and four musicians. Of these, the dancer on the left is basically intact apart from decay in the right hand. Her hair is in a long bun. She wears a short costume with a furled plant design and a long red skirt. Her shoes have high tips and there is a silk scarf draped across her left shoulder. With one end tucked into the front of her jacket, she is lightly clasping the edge of the scarf with her left hand in a dainty pose. Both her right hand and the other end of the scarf have disintegrated. Some people think however that the right arm was held behind her back. The other part of the scarf hangs behind her shoulder (see fig. 60). This silk picture of a dancer unearthed in Xinjiang is the same in dress and style of dancing pose as Han dancers

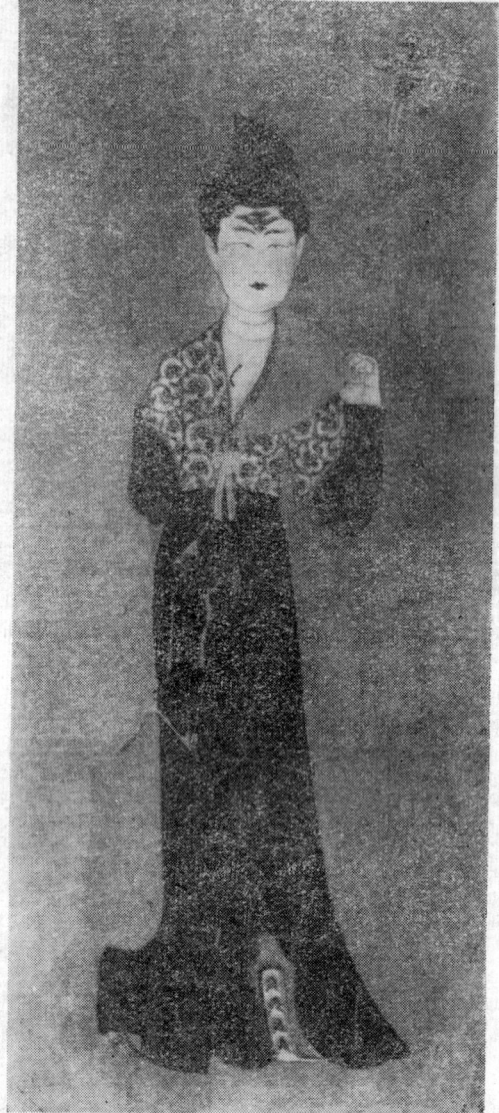

60. One of the Tang music and dance screens (silk painting). Unearthed in Xinjiang.

from the Central Plains area. Evidently there was frequent exchange of dance between the Han people and national minorities under the Tang. Their influence on and assimilation of things from each other are borne out by history.

Though based on tradition, dance in the Tang was boldly innovative, embracing many national folk dances and those brought from abroad. Just as Lu Xun (1881-1936) said, "Although the Han and Tang dynasties also had border troubles, there was nevertheless a great breadth of vision. The people had the confidence not to end up enslaved to other nations, or else the thought did not even occur to them for whenever they adopted anything from abroad it was as if they had taken it prisoner. They did with it as they liked regardless!" ("Thoughts on Looking in a Mirror" in *The Grave*). The wording of this passage penetrates to the very core of the reason for the liberalness with which Tang art absorbed everything. The same applied to dance then too. Given conditions which were politically stable for a fairly long period underpinned by a reasonably prosperous society and economy, conditions conductive to an extensive incorporation of dance from within and without the country were brought about. All these favourable factors were used to full effect in greatly enriching and improving the artistic level of dance itself. A golden age for the development of dance in Chinese feudal society was created.

In A.D. 755 after the "An and Shi Disturbances"* the powerful Tang Dynasty gradually declined. Due to the constant ravages of war, the economy suffered greatly so the court song and dance institutions were reduced substantially. Many of the musicians and dancers who had been rigorously trained were dispersed amongst the populace to play a dynamic role in the subsequent development of folk song and dance.

---

* In 755 A.D., a regional military governor called An Lushan raised troops in armed rebellion at Fanyang (modern Beijing). After his death, his lieutenant Shi Siming carried on the fight against the Tang which was not put down by government troops until A.D. 763. This armed rebellion is known in history as the "An and Shi Disturbances".

CHAPTER SEVEN

Song Folk Dance and "Dance Troupes"

The Five Dynasties and Ten Kingdoms lasting from A.D. 907 to A.D. 979 were a continuation and extension of the separate states set up by military governors at the end of the Tang. Production was severely damaged by the social unrest.

Most of China was unified in A.D. 960 when the Northern Song was established. The Qidan, a national minority in the Northeast of China, founded the Liao and the Dangxiang Qiang, a clan from the Northwest, the Western Xia, thus leading to a long period of confrontation with the Northern Song. The Liao and Western Xia slave-owning classes were constantly waging wars of depradation which brought much pain and suffering to people of all nationalities. In A.D. 1127, the Northern Song was destroyed by a regime set up by the Nüzhen clan which had arisen in the North of China —the Tartars (Kin). Part of the Song court fled south to found their own small dynastic enclave at Lin'an (modern Hangzhou in Zhejiang)—the Southern Song.

During both the Northern and Southern Song, many heavily populated cities with advanced communications came into existence as a result of the development of agriculture, handicrafts and commerce as well as expanded foreign trade. Along with the flourishing of the city economy and popularity of the guild system, folk dance and other performing arts greatly expanded. In the Northern Song capital of Bianliang (now Kaifeng, Henan) and the Southern Song equivalent at Lin'an there were many "Wazi" (like Tianqiao and Changdian in Beijing before Liberation). A series of rings were fenced off in these "Wazi". Known as Goulan they were special venues for the staging of various skills. The setting up of the "Wazi" and "Goulan" gave a definite boost to the upkeep of artists as well as to the transmission and improvement of skills.

There were a large number of "Wazi" at Bianliang in the Northern Song—more than 50 Goulan large and small. The biggest could hold several thousand people and there was always a good audience whatever the weather.

Lin'an under the Southern Song had more than 20 Wazi inside and outside the town. The largest with 13 Goulan was at Beiwa which meant there were 13 venues putting on shows at the same time. Besides these, there were also performing artists earning a living on the streets and squares.

All kinds of skills were performed at the Wazi, it really was a case of "a great display of a variety of acts". There were poetic dramas set to music, acrobatics, various kinds of story-telling, double comic acts, shadow theatre, puppets, free form music, all sorts of musical acts, wrestling and various dances.

"Wuxuan" referred to performances of dance alone. The pirouette was probably the staple dancing technique then so dance pieces were generally thus named as Wuxuan literally meant "to dance wheeling". Even today various turning movements are still important components of basic dance work. Zhang Zhennu was a famous exponent of the genre under the Northern Song. The institution for music and dance then — the Jiaofang — listed the following styles "Wuxuan", "poetic dramas", "Song and Clapper", and "Pipa". Each "style" had a chief and each department a department head who led the professional performers under them in their various fields.

"Dance to Foreign Music" was a performance of national minority dance, evidence of the state of song and dance exchange between the Han and minority nationalities. Zhang Yuxi was a famous performer in this style at Lin'an during the Southern Song.

The Song "Acting the Big Head" was in the same tradition as the "Monk with a Big Head" widespread in the Yuan (1271-1368) Ming (1368-1644) and Qing dynasties. The *Miscellaneous Poems for New Year* compiled by Wu Xilin mentions that "(The Monk) Mingyue Converts Liu Cui to Buddhism" occurs in the "Hundred Works" of the Yuan and in Ming "poetic dramas" which both adopted this folk dance form. It was generally performed in the streets at the Lantern Festival. "Children of the Mountain Spirit dance up, all wearing large false heads decorated with coloured drawings. Hence the name, the Monk with a Big Head", and the motto on the lanterns "Monks with Big Heads Fill the Streets". The "Dry Boat Religious Festival Show" (see fig. 61, top right) is depicted in the Qing painting *A Religious Festival in Beijing*. Behind the "Dry Boat" are three figures wearing large heads. There is a man carrying a horsetail whisk dressed as a monk and a woman wearing a gown. Her left hand is behind her back with a fan in it and the right one is holding a handkerchief over her mouth. Another man is a short tunic stands with his hands on his hips. It is very probably the popular Qing "Monk with a Big Head Dallies with Liu Cui". The item "Paddling a Dry Boat" is being performed and these three people are standing at the back as if waiting their turn to perform. This type of popular dance tradition was carried on amongst the populace. After Liberation, dancers and choreographers used such traditional dance forms in children's dance arrangements like the "Big-Headed Children". The children's group dance from the dance drama "Precious Lotus Lamp" took the same form and proved very popular.

The "Flower Drum" has been handed down until the present day as one of the best liked dance forms. Although it existed by name in the Song, no detailed accounts of how it was performed have come to light.

All kinds of Flower Drum dance were performed throughout China. Before Liberation when poor people from the area of Shandong left their homes to escape famine, they often earned their living by performing the Flower Drum. They would sing while playing. There were 12 ways of striking the drum characterized by the wheeling flourishes. The tassels on the drumsticks were used in concert to hit the drum, a complicated skill, while the dancing poses were bold and unconstrained. After Liberation, dancers developed and improved on the form of the dance in a compilation called the "Flower Drum Dance" which was warmly received in China as well as being popular on foreign tours. The "Fengyang Flower Drum" from Anhui was performed by a man and a woman. One played a small gong, the other the Flower Drum as they sang and danced. Many forms of Flower Drum come from Shanxi. They are divided into the High Drum (the drum hangs in front of the chest), Low Drum (the drum is at the waist), Multi-Drum (drums hanging from waist, chest and shoulder are beaten in turn during the dance). A local folk saying describes the "Flower Drum Dance": "Hands hit the drum, feet beat the gong, the shaking of the head is the cymbals...."

Lifting the head, sticking out the chest with both feet moving, gestures, gong and drum together combined." The dancing was closely linked to the beat of the music. Rich in its diversity and with a long history, the "Flower Drum Dance" is one of the many forms of Chinese drum dance.

The "Dance of the Sabre" and "Dance of the Chopper" both evolved from martial arts. There are records of Sabre Dances as early as the Han. In the Tang it was a spectacular dance number. Today as well, there are still beautiful sabre dances included in some traditional opera programmes such as the "Xiang Yu Parts with His Concubine" in Beijing opera. Swordsmanship and knife play from martial arts have preserved many bold and vigorous dancing poses of great beauty too.

In his book *Memories of the Eastern Capital*, Meng Yuanlao of the Southern Song gives a fairly clear account of dance performances at "Wazi" of the Song time.

For the "Tribal Shield Dance", the orchestra played "Qinjia Nongling". More than 100 warriors "in colourful short costumes" appeared on stage. In front came a man wielding a flag. Those behind carried pheasant tails, tribal shields and wooden swords. They formed up in ranks to make various group formations. Afterwards they stood grouped in the semi-circular "Crescent Moon Battle Array". The orchestra struck up with the "Command for Tribal Shields". Two people broke rank to dance together making stabbing movements at each other. "One of them would lunge forward, and the other fall prostrate (to show he had been hit and fallen to the ground)".

They then went off stage. Half a dozen or so pairs of performers came on, with spears versus shields or swords versus shields. The dance derived from ancient battle life. Possibly it was a continuation of the even older "Shield and Axe Dance" and was in the same tradition as the "Shield Dance" and "Cane Shield Dance" which are still popular among the people today.

The "Dance Judgement" was in fact the "Dance of Zhong Kui". The story goes that Zhong Kui was of great learning and came first in the Imperial Examinations. However, merely because he looked ugly the Emperor disqualified him. In a fury, Zhong Kui knocked his head on the wall and killed himself. After his death the Emperor of Heaven made him "General for Exorcising Evil". This legend reflected ordinary people's dissatisfaction with the exam system and their sympathy for Zhong Kui. Wen Tingjun, a poet in the Tang, was also very learned but ugly. He was nicknamed Wen Zhongkui so clearly this legend was already in existence during the Tang. Zhong Kui in the Song "Dance Judgement" wore a mask and false beard. Dressed in a green robe and boots, he held bamboo slips (used for writing on in ancient times) as he appeared on stage. Obviously there was already a set form for the character Zhong Kui then. A man in the wings played a small gong as Zhong Kui came on and hit it in time to the dance steps.

"Acting Zhong Kui" was one of the Ming poetic dramas and "Zhong Kui Marries Off His Sister" has been handed down from the early Qing until the present day. It tells how Zhong Kui thought about his sister all alone with no one to help her after his death. Taking several small devils with him he went in person to marry her off. It is a song and dance drama with an interesting layout. The figure of Zhong Kui, ugly to look at but warm at heart, and the five mischievous little devils are portrayed with great success. The dancing proceeds in step with the contents of the songs in a beautiful combination of highly skilled and difficult dance movements. The phrasing is clear and the rhythm distinct. At each pause, new and interesting scenarios can appear forming beautiful tableaux which create a lively stage atmosphere. It is an opera piece with a strong dance flavour.

"Flapping the Flag" was performed in the Song by someone in a red headscarf who carried two white flags and "danced with leaps and whirls". The term "Flapping the Flag" survives to this day in traditional opera. Generally it is used in stirring scenes of fighting when the floating and furling of the flag is closely co-ordinated with tumbling, jumping and rolling movements. An ingenious combination of martial arts and dance, when flawlessly executed the effect is as if the swiftly dancing performer and the floating flag are almost one and the same thing. The flag is generally no longer white but light green or blue for naval battles to represent the water; and often red for land battles to heighten the aura of fierce fighting.

Many of the song and dance pieces performed at the Wazi of the Song Dynasty were dance or mainly in the dance genre. However, from the point of view of all the performing arts, the new poetic dramas were "the standard thing"—the most welcome and appreciated by people. There was a wide variety of other types such as storytelling or ballad-singing which were also widespread.

There was a large number of amateur dance performers common in the Song which had been passed on from generation to generation. On festival days each village and city guild had its own folk dance troupe — sometimes called a "Shehuo" (from the name of a festival at the beginning of Spring). However this so called dance troupe did not just perform song and dance but also included performances of various skills. Folk dance troupes of the Song were very similar to the shows staged at religious festivals during the Qing and more or less the same as the "Floral Groups" still common in Hebei and other places. They were integrated performing groups which used to parade the streets. Included were age-old items of folk dance or pieces with a strong element of dance. We will first identify and then describe them.

One of the Song folk dance numbers was "Catching Butterflies" which together with other folk dances such as the "Dancing Dragon Lantern" also figured in the Qing seasonal dramas. It portrayed children playing and continued as a popular tradition right up until after Liberation. A group of girls held fans and a boy carried a brightly decorated rattan cane with a paper butterfly tied on top. The "butterfly" fluttered round hovering in the air as the fans encircled it dancing to and fro trying to catch it. It had a great deal of gusto. After Liberation, the show "Picking Tea and Catching Butterflies", an arrangement by Chinese dancers based on such folk dances, was warmly received and praised by both Chinese and foreign audiences.

The Tartars were an ancient Chinese nationality which still exists today. They first crop up in records from the Tang and were originally a tribe under the rule of the Turks. The "Tartar Dance" was their national folk dance. It used to be performed at Lin'an during the Southern Song being one and the same as the "Dance to Foreign Music" mentioned earlier — clear proof of cultural contacts between the Han and national minorities.

Accounts about the "Dry Boat" had existed in the Tang Dynasty. During the Song, Fan Chengda wrote the line "From afar the Dry Boats look as if they are floating" in a poem. The poet added the note that "Rowing the Dry Boat is the name for a dance performed on a narrow piece of ground on dry land like the boat race". Rowing Dragon Boats on the rivers was an ancient Chinese custom, the Song "Dry Dragon Boat" was a copy of such activities on dry land. From a distance, the boats looked as if they were floating in water. The section "Racing Dry Boats" at the Lantern

Festival in the Qing *Notes on the Seasons at Yanjing* states that "Racing Dry Boats was when village lads dressed up as girls and moved cloth boats about by hand as they sang street songs. It was meant to be an imitation of boating on the lake to pick lotuses ... and went on until the busy season when they stopped and returned to ploughing." Such was the scene at a performance of "Racing Dry Boats" at the rural Lantern Festival during the Qing. The picture of the "Dry Boat Show" in the Qing painting *A Religious Festival in Beijing* has a girl "sitting" in a "cloth boat". In stage costume and makeup, she is holding a fan in her right hand. A boatman with makeup on holds a bamboo pole as if punting the boat along. To one side are four accompanists — one with a large drum on his back, another beating it and the last two clashing cymbals (see fig. 61, bottom right). It is more or less the same as the present-day "Racing Dry Boats" common among the people. In modern performances a female character has a cloth boat tied to her waist. It covers her legs and feet so she looks as if she is sitting in it. A man holds an oar in a rowing position. Sometimes the girl performs smooth dance-steps to represent the boat being rowed across the water. At others, the two of them face each other to depict the rocking of the boat in the water by a co-ordination of rising and falling movements as they sing and dance. This age-old yet fresh and lively folk dance can still be seen today in processions on festival days.

How the "Bamboo Horse" in Song folk troupes was performed is not quite clear. However in the section entitled "A Miscellany of Plays Throughout the Year" in the Qing *Seasonal Festivities in the Imperial*

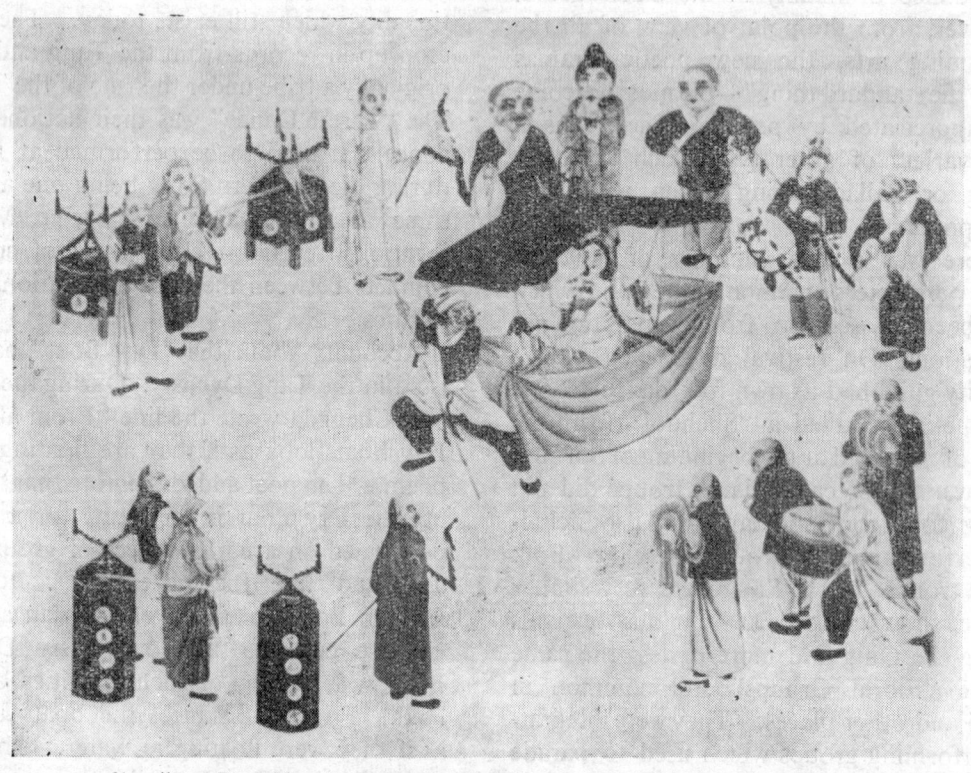

61. "Dry Boat Show" in the Qing painting *A Religious Festival in Beijing*.

Capital, there are records about "Riding the Bamboo Horse". It was a common folk dance in several areas of China and featured a prop shaped like a horse in two sections, the head and tail, which was tied to the waist of the dancer. The dancer appeared to be on horseback as he performed various actions such as the horse ambling along, galloping or jumping. The performer sang songs at the same time as dancing. There is a girl in the "Dry Boat Religious Festival Show" from the Qing painting *A Religious Festival in Beijing*. She has a horse's head and tail tied to her waist and a whip in her left hand. To the left, a clown also holding a whip stands behind the "Dry Boat". He is tilting his head towards her (see fig. 61, top right). They are both performers in "Racing the Bamboo Horse" who are waiting to go on stage. It is similar in form to the well-known folk dances "Racing a Donkey" and "Racing the Bamboo Horse" from the early years of Liberation.

Bao Lao was the name for a character in puppet plays who led the dancing as well as for a comic dance in the folk dance troupes. The "Puppet Poem" by Yang Danian of the Song period says, "Bao Lao made fun of Guo Lang before the audience for having flicked his sleeves in a sloppy manner; but when he was asked to dance at a banquet, he thought it would be better to get Jue Lang to toss his sleeves." As can be seen Bao Lao and Guo Lang were comic characters in puppet shows. According to a passage on "Puppets" in the *Miscellaneous Notes from the Board of Music*, "Guo Lang leads the singing and dancing. He is bald and good at the comic role in the villages they call Guo Lang. He has to be top of the bill at shows." Guo Lang led the dancing in Tang puppet shows, and his part must have been of a similar type to Bao Lao's as they are both mentioned together. *Tales of the Old Capital*, an account of local conditions and customs in the Southern Song capital of Lin'an, says that puppets dancing the "Bao Lao" was included on the programme at the Song court on the fifth day of the first month. This would have been a puppet performance of the "Bao Lao Dance". The version in Song folk dance troupes seems then to have been people imitating the dance in puppet shows. The public very much enjoyed watching such comic dances on festival days. Another work recording cultural activities and entertainments for citizens at Lin'an, the *Record of Prosperity by the Old Man of the West Lake*, says that, "the Bao Lao from Fujian has more than thirty people in a company. The one from Sichuan more than a hundred". It is probably referring to Bao Lao dance troupes with a local flavour or else dance troupes organized by "Associations of Fellow Townsmen" for people from Fujian and Sichuan living at Lin'an.

"Ten Scholars" was included in Song dance troupe programmes possibly to satirize those who bought the post of "scholar" for money. The *Collection of Poems of Zhang Tuian* contains the line "the young boy flicks his sleeves like a scholar, the elder girl laughs to see him making mischief" — the comic effect of a child swishing his sleeves in imitation of a scholar. In the way it ridicules the feudal ruling class the Song "Ten Scholars" is similar to "Carrying the Box" from the Qing *A Religious Festival in Beijing* (see fig. 62). This was when an official with his nose comically whitened with powder was carried round in procession. On the way people pretended to block the route to lodge complaints, possibly they were all to expose "official" wrongdoings. Thus the "Popular Works from Beiping" says: "In carrying the box the official can have great fun, he shields himself with an open umbrella ... afraid that those in the know will lodge complaints. According to a survey by members of the Shandong Song and Dance Troupe, before Liberation the

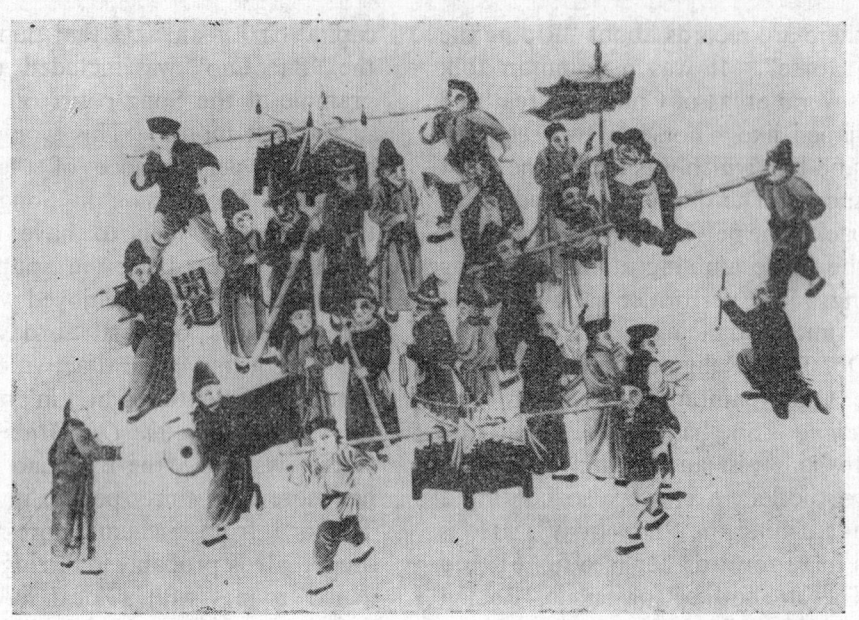

62. "Carrying the Box" in the Qing painting *A Religious Festival in Beijing*.

Yangge troupe in the Liaocheng area of Shandong included a "Carrying". That too involved carrying someone "who had been promoted" (an official) wearing a half face mask which left his nose and mouth exposed. For up to three days the local county officials could be sworn at without being punished. The people made clever use of folk song and dance to expose and ridicule the darkness of the reactionary ruling classes.

"Village Music" was a folk song and dance with a strong local flavour which depicted agricultural life. The Song poet Fan Chengda in a poem describing the marvellous scene at a performance of "Village Music" by a folk company during the Lantern Festival wrote the line, "People in village rain capes and hats". Apparently when "Village Music" was put on, performers had to dress up as peasants by wearing palm-bark rain capes and straw hats.

There is as yet no first hand record of how "Village Music" was performed in the Yuan. However there is a piece in the Yuan poetic drama "Liu Xuande Walks Drunk to the Yellow Crane Pavilion" where a fat girl and boy imitate songs and dances depicting agricultural work from shows at Lantern Festivals. To the tune of "Daodaoling" they sing of "The bald girl at the well, cranking on the windlass clink clink clink"; "the fat blind girl hulling rice on the threshing floor chonk chonk chonk"; "the servants carrying whips which whistle swish swish swish"; "the ox-herd riding backwards on the water buffalo singing ya ya ya". It can be inferred that this song and dance passage with its depictions of rural working life such as drawing water, hulling rice and herding oxen was very probably a continuation and development of the Song "Village Music".

Some changes had taken place in "Village Music" by the time it was handed down to the Qing. *Miscellaneous Poems for New Year* written by Wu Xiqi records that the "Yangge" was "Village Music" from the Southern Song Lantern Festivals. Characters included monks, young gentlemen, Flower Drum players, Lahua girls (editor's note: a female role in Yangge troupes was called "Lahua", also the name for a form of Yangge dance), villagers, fishermen's wives and people playing travelling salesmen. They crowded the lantern hung streets making the onlookers laugh. From this brief account we can tell that much of the repertoire from Song folk dance troupes had been carried on into the Qing. They were no longer called "Dancing Troupes" but "Yangge" (troupes). The Qing Yangge and the Song "Village Music" were linked by inheritance. The close ties folk dance had with people's lives and work gave it a broad popular base and stubborn vitality. As a result it could continue to spread and improve during the long period of unrest.

Folk dances in the Song were many and varied. They gave lively depictions of all kinds of people in scenes from life. This rich vitality was very different from the Tang dances which portrayed simple sentiments or styles.

The Song court "Troupe Dances" were sequels to and developments of the Tang "Yan Music". Although pieces included such as "Mulberry Branch", "Sabre Dance", "Tartar Prancing", "Huntuo" and "Rainbow-Coloured Clothes" and all continued under Tang dance names, there had already been changes in format. They were mainly performed when ceremonies were held at court. "Fine words" of culogy (an expression of good wishes at the start of the piece) or songs were added for these performances.

The country became weaker during the late Northern Song and the Southern Song so that the court could no longer maintain large institutions for music and dance. Whenever there were big court celebrations artists were temporarily hired from amongst the populace to take part in performances. *Tales of the Old Capital* states that during the Qiandao and Chunxi periods of the Southern Song (1165-1189), large numbers of temporarily hired people were on the lists of artists drawn up by the Department of Music at the Jiaofang.

The Song were heirs to the large song and dance ceremonies of the Tang which were developed and altered a little. Not simply performances of dance alone they were interleaved with sections relating or portraying the story of a character. The "Sabre Dance" described by Shi Hao of the Song is given here as an example to show how large song and dance ceremonies were performed then.

To begin, a pair of dancers stood on a mat and the "Bamboo Pole" (like a compère) said a small piece (similar to the explanation before a performance).

Next the two of them spoke some lines and exchanged a few words with the "Bamboo Pole".

The music ensemble sang the quick tempoed "Sabre" dance music as the pair of dancers performed the piece.

Both dancers sang "Reveille on a Frosty Day".

The ensemble sang the tune again and the fast rhythmed "Sabre" dance piece was performed once more.

The dance finished, the dancers stood apart on either side.

Two more people wearing Han Dynasty costumes came on stage and sat opposite each other. Drink and fruit were set on a table. The "Bamboo Pole" told the story of the banquet at Hongmen. It is about Liu Bang (i.e. the Han Emperor Gaozu) taking the Qin capital Xianyang in A.D. 206 and then sending soldiers to guard the Hangu Pass. A little later Xiang Yu attacked at the head of a large 400,000-strong army. He entered Hongmen (east of modern Lintong in Shaanxi) and made ready to wipe out Liu Bang. Through the mediation of Xiang Yu's uncle, Liu Bang came in person to Hongmen to meet Xiang Yu. At the banquet, an advisor called Fan Zeng asked Xiang Zhuang to perform the "Sabre Dance".

He hoped to take advantage of the opportunity to assassinate Liu Bang. Xiang Yu's uncle drew his sword and danced as well frequently shielding Liu Bang with his body. Only when the Han general Fan Kuai finally rushed in fully armed was Liu Bang able to make good his escape.

In the section where the music ensemble sang the melody and the swift tempoed "Sabre" piece was performed, the dancer on the left went onto the mat to dance gesturing as if trying to stab the character dressed in Han costume (playing Liu Bang). Another dancer came on stage drawing closer as he danced and made motions as if to protect the man in Han dress. At the close, the dancers and the character in Han costume drew back.

Next two people in Tang dress came on and sat opposite each other. On the table were brushes, inkstone and paper.

One of the dancers had changed into woman's clothes and stood on the mat. The "Bamboo Pole" told the story of how the Tang calligrapher Zhang Xu made great progress in his cursive script after watching Gongsun dance the "Sabre". He also went on to recount the story of Du Fu writing his famous poem "Watching a Pupil of Gongsun in the Sabre Dance" after seeing a performance.

The music ensemble sang the "Sabre" dance music while the dancers performed "graceful dance actions like wriggling dragons and snakes".

The couple in Tang dress rose. The two dancers — a man (playing Xiang Yu's uncle from the Han) and a woman (in the part of Gongsun from the Tang) performed a pas de deux as the last section of the "Sabre" piece. The dance finished. The "Bamboo Pole" read poems praising Xiang Yu's

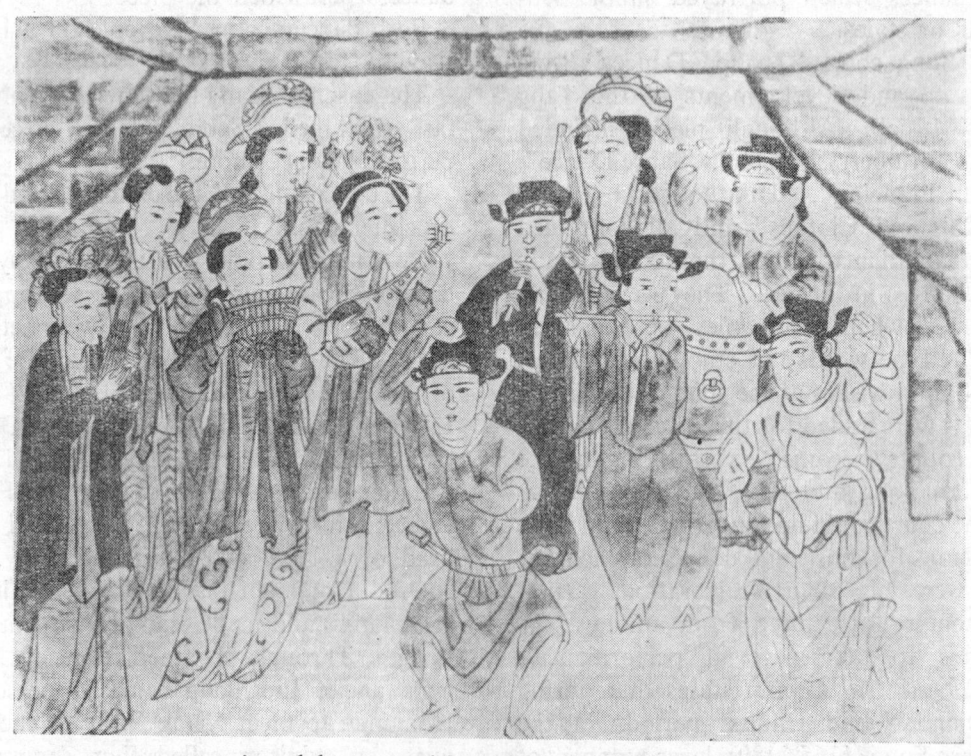

63. A music and dance mural from Zhao Daweng's tomb of the Song. Unearthed at Yuxian, Henan.

uncle and Gongsun and announced the piece had ended. The way in which this show brought together two historical characters separated by several hundred years was romantic in the extreme.

As can be seen from the examples above large song and dance ceremonies in the Song were no longer just performances of dance. Sections depicting stories, sometimes in song, were mixed in. The art of traditional opera gradually took shape during this process of development.

Though Song folk dance did flourish it was mostly as a mass activity on festival days. Poetic drama was paramount within the realm of performing arts. In his *A Consideration of Song and Yuan Traditional Opera* the modern scholar Wang Guowei (1877-1927) researched in great detail those sections from official scripts of poetic drama contained in the Song *Tales of the Old Capital*. There were 280 in all, those for large ceremonies accounting for 103. This proves that poetic dramas absorbed a lot from song and dance acts.

Moreover the historical background to the close connection between dance and traditional opera during the course of their development is also evident from music and dance murals uncovered in Song and Liao (A.D. 916-1125) tombs. One was uncovered at Yuxian County, Henan in Zhao Daweng's tomb which dates from A.D. 1099 under the Song. The dancer in the middle wears a headscarf and long belted robe. His legs are in the "riding crouched down" pose. His right hand is held above his head while the left hand is bent in front of his chest. Ten musicians with pipes, strings and percussion at the ready surround the dancers at the back (see fig. 63). On the east wall of the Liao coffin chamber (A.D. 1116) unearthed at Xuanhua in Hebei was a "Picture of Free Form Music". A squat dancer wearing a headscarf, belted gown and boots stands in the middle of a full orchestra of 11 people. He is clasping his elbows at an angle in front of his chest. The upper part of his body tilts to the right as he bends over with his left leg taking the weight. The right heel is touching the ground with the sole of the foot pointed upwards as he gracefully dances (see fig. 64). The figures of dancers in the two murals above are very similar in both dress and form to dances from traditional opera in later generations.

The music and dance scene on a screen with Buddhist religious paintings from the Song murals in Cavern No. 61 at the Mogao Caves, Dunhuang, breathes with life. Three musicians sit to one side playing an accompaniment while a dancing girl, her hair in a tall bun and wearing a long skirt gathered at the waist, dances with her long sleeves trailing behind her (see fig. 65). The dancing pose is close in both form and style

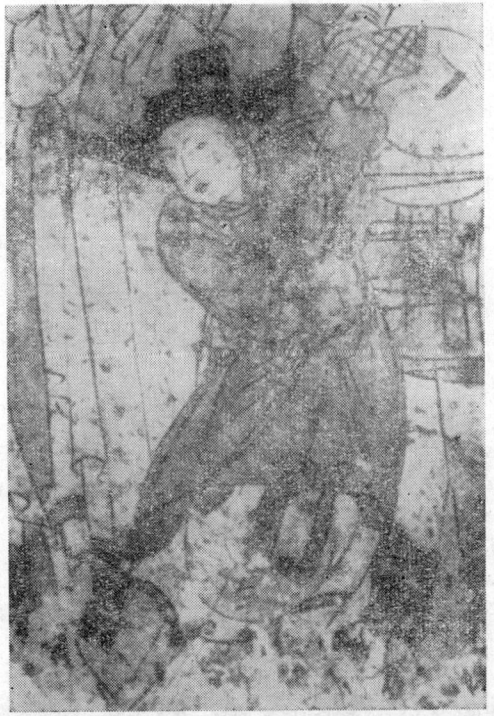

64. Dance in a "Picture of Free Form Music" on a mural from a Liao coffin chamber (detail). Unearthed in Xuanhua, Hebei.

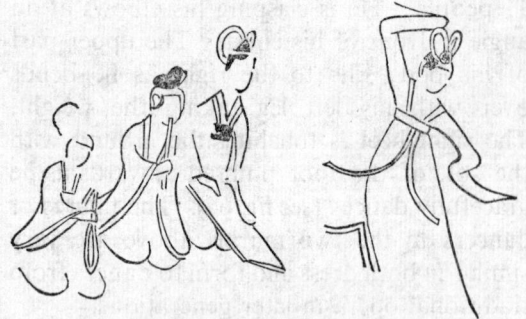

65. Copy of part of a Song mural of music and dance at Cavern No. 61 of the Mogao Caves in Dunhuang.

to those in Han stone reliefs as well as being similar to the "Shaking of One Sleeve" in dances from traditional opera. It is clear that a wealth of traditional dance has indeed been preserved in Chinese classical opera.

The Northern and Southern Song were periods when complex class and national contradictions were at breaking point. The cruel economic exploitation and political suppression of working people by the ruling classes forced the peasants to rise up and revolt in continual peasant rebellions. The populace were fed up with the greed, violence and debauched life of the ruling classes and needed a new art form to be created. It was to express such complex thoughts and feelings that the art of traditional opera with its many means of expression suited to meet this need arose and developed on the basis of life in the cities where there were large audiences. From the Song and Yuan up until the Qing all kinds of traditional opera continued to arise and proved to be the most popular form of art throughout that period.

CHAPTER EIGHT

Dance and Traditional Opera During the Ming and Qing Dynasties

The Ming was the feudal dynasty founded in 1368 after a peasant revolt at the end of the Yuan.

A peasant rebel army led by Li Zicheng entered the capital at Beijing in 1644 and overthrew the reign of the Ming Dynasty. In the same year the Qing army, invited across the pass into China by Wu Sangui, set up the Qing Dynasty.

The Ming and Qing dynasties gradually entered upon the final stage of Chinese feudal society. From the middle of the Ming onwards, feudal society bore the seeds of capitalism within itself. A thriving city life spurred on a boom in such arts as traditional opera, singing and story telling. With the rise of traditional opera, performances of dances by themselves were rarely seen. However, dance which had merged together with traditional opera continued developing and improving to form a fairly comprehensive training and performing system. It thus preserved the rich and splendid tradition of classical dance. At the same time the growth of new economic factors influenced social life and the development of the arts as well as people's way of thinking. Democratic thought opposed to feudalism and autocracy made headway and came to be reflected more and more clearly in works of art such as traditional opera, novels and folk songs and dances. To control peoples' thinking, the ruling class went even further in its destruction, prohibition and denigration of the arts. The increasing severity of the feudal ethical code during this period meant women were no longer able to take part in folk dances. The female roles were mostly played by men which was a definite hindrance to the development of dance.

During the Yuan, Ming and Qing dynasties the growing intensity of both class and national contradictions spurred people on in their search for an artistic form which showed more directly the harshness of their lives and their spirit of resistance. It was rather difficult for song and dance alone to meet these requirements whereas the art of traditional opera was suitable. As a result, traditional opera grew in popularity, dance gradually merging with it to form a component part of such performances. Pure dance then rarely existed as an independent performing art apart from some which still circulated amongst the populace.

Dance in Traditional Opera

From the Song and Yuan onwards, traditional opera gradually replaced song and dance which had been most prominent in the Sui and Tang dynasties to become a highly popular form of performing art.

Chinese traditional opera is a composite performing art, which developed out of the legacy of many different art forms from previous dynasties. A variety of genres such as literature, drama, music, dance, fine art, martial arts and acrobatics are cleverly brought together in depictions of the rich tapestry of life and the characters of different types of people which are unfolded in a complex plot. Dance is an important component in traditional opera. It inherited the classical song and dance of previous dynasties while absorbing a large number of folk genres from various places. Thus a wealth of traditional dances are preserved in opera. Some merged with the choreography and postures in theatrical performances, others being inserted fairly intact as dance passages.

The opera in vogue during the Ming — the poetic drama — developed from Southern Drama. It broke through the constraints of form in the Yuan poetic dramas in which one person sang for all four acts. Every character was now able to sing and do some performing. Generally the form of presentation was similar to present-day traditional opera except that the librettos then were tediously long. No specific records have emerged as to how the dances were arranged within these poetic dramas. We can only hazard a guess from fragmentary accounts.

Recollections of Tao An, a work by Zhang Dai at the end of the Ming, gives an accurate account of the training for operatic artists then and of dance scenes in some pieces. It says that when Zhu Yunxia instructed actresses he "first taught zither, *pipa, tiqin, xianzi* (all string instruments), *shao* (a wind instrument), drum and pipes, singing and dancing before she taught acting". As can be seen, the training for the performers was quite comprehensive. They had to understand music, learn to play as well as study song and dance. This all round training meant the song and dance scenes they staged were of a moving beauty: "In the Xi Shi song and dance, five people danced together, slowly bearing their long sleeves which encircled their bodies like hoops. They would touch the ground while the dancers whirl gracefully round and round." This would have been impossible without rigorous physical training. The same book tells of the "Actress Liu Huiji". "For example: 'The Tang Emperor Minghuang Tours the Palace on the Moon'... a clap of thunder and the black curtain is suddenly drawn back to reveal the round orb of a moon, multi-coloured clouds of dyed wool everywhere. In the middle sits Changyi (Chang'e), Wu Gang, the cassia tree, the white rabbit grinding medicine in a mortar. Veiled in thin silk cloth, several lamps are lit inside as bright as the moon. The colour is bluish like early dawn. Cloth is strung here and there to form hills and caves, a magical realm — you forget it is a play. There are also dances with lamps, a score or so of people each carrying one, flickering to and fro, wonders at every turn." They actually had such brilliant stage scenery and lighting 300 or 400 years ago. Folk Lantern Dances were also incorporated into performances of traditional opera to great theatrical effect.

Kunqu Opera popular in the Ming and Qing went even further in its amalgamation of dance with the singing and acting performances. It is apparent from old traditionnal pieces that Kunqu Opera was an integration of song and dance which placed equal stress on the singing and acting. The poetic drama "Peony Pavilion" by the Ming dramatist Tang Xianzu (1550-1616) is a romantic classic of Chinese theatre. The story concerns Du Liniang, the daughter of the prefect at Nan'an, who went strolling in the garden with her maid servant for something to do. Tired from walking, she took a nap and fell in love with a scholar she dreamt of — Liu Mengmei. Upon waking Du Liniang pined away with sorrow. Three years later Liu Mengmei went on convalescence to Nan'an and found a self-portrait by Du Liniang. He fell deeply in love with her. She sensed it and came back to life. They finally became man and wife. One of the scenes in this work "A Startling Dream During a Stroll in the Garden" is a traditional Kunqu Opera piece. Through the various forms used — beauty and gentleness, deep love and affection and singing together with dancing — the yearning of a cloistered young girl for a free and happy love life is portrayed in a beautiful yet lively way. Each phrase in the singing is accompanied by dance movements which fit in with the meaning of the words. The combination of movements is well ordered. Both characters worked well with each other often forming beautiful scenarios. When Du Liniang meets Liu Mengmei in her dream there is a group dance scene in which the Flower God piles up flowers. The traditional manner of presentation makes use of forms from folk dance troupes and Lantern Dances. It is a song and dance show with a fairly complete structure.

There is a scene in the "Tale of the Sword" by Li Kaixian of the Ming entitled "Lin Chong Flees by Night". It describes the story of how the hero Lin Chong kills his persecutors and flees by night to the rebel army at Liangshan Marsh. The choreography for the piece is highly skilled and vivid including evocative dancing poses of great strength. Others such as "Thinking of Worldly Things" which depicts a young nun who longs for lay life and runs away from the convent on a mountain and "Zhong Kui Marries Off His Sister" are all pieces from the traditional Kunqu repertoire which are strongly dance oriented.

Compositions for Wind and Percussion from Kunqu Opera edited by our contemporary Gao Buyun includes a category for "dance compositions" namely accompanying music for dances in this kind of opera. Both "Parasol Tree Rain", a poetic drama by the Yuan dramatist Bai Pu (1226-?) and the Kunqu Opera "The Palace of Eternal Youth", an arrangement of the famous work by the Qing dramatist Hong Sheng (1645-1704), portray the love and lives of the Tang Emperor Minghuang and Lady Yang. They also both include details of Lady Yang's "Tray Dance", though the score is not the same. The late Mei Lanfang, the famous Beijing Opera artiste, thought that Kunqu Opera "has all the various types of body postures, both dainty and demanding, set out in the librettos, the meaning of whatever is being sung about has to be related to the audience through the actions. So in terms of the integration of song and dance with equal stress being laid on both singing and acting, Kunqu Opera is unsurpassed".

Opera artists have created fairly comprehensive performing and training methods through practice of their art over a long period of time and their own unrelenting research. They have produced a rich and varied choreography with great impact as well as all kinds of performing styles. Such highly wrought and stylized dance movements have continued to develop and evolve in the process of being handed down over the years. Study and research into dance movements in traditional opera are of great significance for the continuation and further improvement of the Chinese dance tradition.

Small Folk Song and Dance Shows

Influenced by the traditional operatic arts, folk song and dance from various areas gradually developed into many small song and dance shows during the Qing. An example is the Flower Drum Show which circulated widely in Hunan, Hubei, Anhui and Jiangsu and had evolved from folk song and dance such as the "Local Flower Drum" and "Flower Lantern". In the book *Notes from Mingzhai* written by Zhu Lian who lived during the Qianlong and Jiaqing periods (1736-1820) of the Qing it says that, "There have been many changes in the Flower Drum Show during the 30 years it has been handed down. First it was performed by males and then females. It was performed during the day and then by night. It started in the countryside and was continued in the towns. Initially popular amongst country folk, it was later taken up by the young men about town". The speed with which the Flower Drum Show developed and the extent of its popularity is evident.

The Tea Picking Show developed from the folk song and dance, "Tea Picking Lantern". Judging by the fact there was already a decree strictly forbidding performances of "Tea Picking" in the Qing, this small song and dance show was already very popular then. According to surveys by opera and music researchers since Liberation, the precursor of the Tea Picking Show at Nanchang, Jiangxi, was a folk song and dance called the "Tea Lantern Song", the most popular item in which was "Tea Picking in Twelve Months". Twelve people carrying flower lanterns dressed as tea picking girls. Each would sing the name of a flower. Such folk dances were already common in Guangdong during the Qing. Li Diaoyuan who wrote *Notes from Eastern Guangdong* then says, "However, the best is the Tea Picking Song, a custom from Guangdong. On the first month of the year, young lads are dressed up as beautiful women, twelve in a group. They carry flower baskets illuminated by lanterns covered in crimson silk and form into a large ring. They circle round singing and dancing 'Tea Picking in Twelve Months'." So it was a tea picking song and dance acted by children for the Spring Festival. Later the "Tea Lantern Song" evolved into the "Three-Role Group" in which just two or three people performed small shows depicting the lives and loves of working people. It was not until part-time groups had been formed (troupe-members earned a living working in the fields during the busy season and performing when it was slack) that historical dramas or large shows devoted to folktales were performed. The perfectly proportioned Tea Picking Shows from around the time of Liberation only came into being at the very end.

Wuxi Opera from Jiangsu, commonly known as Wuxi rhymed story-telling, was also influenced by the "Tea Picking Lantern". According to what old troupers say, during Xianfeng and Tongzhi periods (1851-1874) of the Qing the "Tea Picking Lantern", a folksong and dance widely popular in the Yangtze delta, was put on in each locality every year at the Spring Festival (Wuxi rhymed story-telling was still sung sat down then). The Wuxi story-tellers absorbed dance movements from the piece and gradually founded Wuxi opera. Calculating from the death of a first generation Wuxi Opera artiste (Xu Abao) at the end of the Tongzhi period of the Qing, this art form would have arisen some time between the years 1851-74.

Other shows such as Ningpo Opera developed out of folk songs and dances like the "Horse Lantern Melody" and the "Field Path Song" from the area of Ningpo in

Zhejiang at the end of the Qing. About the time of the Taiping Heavenly Kingdom, Sizhou Opera evolved from folk songs and dances in Anhui, such as the "Yangge" and "Work Songs". There are many similar examples which will not be given separately here.

It was some time before these small folk song and dance acts, initially amateur performances by working people during the slack season, formed into small touring groups composed of probably seven or eight people. They became deeply rooted in people's lives, pouring out their joys and sorrows, singing of their hopes and spirit of resistance and exposing the dark feudal rule.

The development of certain of these small folk song and dance shows differed. Some progressed to traditional opera forming a variety of small local dramas or else went one stage further and evolved into large operatic genres or merged with other kinds of opera. On the other hand, the original song and dance forms continued to circulate amongst the populace. There are many examples of this. After the Hunan folk song and dance "Local Flower Drum" had developed into the Flower Drum Show, the original folk form was still widespread. Or once the Fujian Tea Picking Show had taken shape, its precursor the "Tea Picking Lantern" continued to circulate. The Flower Lantern Show developed out of a folk song and dance in Yunnan called the "Flower Lantern" which however remained there preserved in its many forms. So after Liberation among the people of Yunnan there was the "Wooden Bench Lantern", in oratorio form, a group song and dance form which performed a variety of "Flower Lantern Dances" as well as the "Flower Lantern" in which a story was related in song with no connection between the choreography and the tale's content. In fact the Yunnan "Flower Lantern" covered almost the whole process of development from song to dance to final evolution into a traditional opera. Moreover, the artistic forms from each stage in its development have been preserved. They exist side by side helping each other forward and developing together. This is a common occurrence in the course of development of folk songs and dances from different areas of China into traditional operas.

Folk Dance

In the Ming and Qing dynasties, performances of dancing by themselves were already uncommon though group dances at festivals were still fairly active.

The 15th day of the first month in the lunar calendar is the traditional Lantern Festival. It was the liveliest day for song and dance in the Ming and Qing just as it had been in the Tang and Song. As shown in accounts of the spectacle at a Lantern Festival in Shaoxing, Zhejiang, from the book *Recollections of Tao An* by Zhao Dai of the Ming: Coloured lanterns of all kinds hung from every house and street. "Besides that there were lion dances, drums, wind and string instruments and singing. Fireworks were let off. It was packed with people, in main streets and twisting alleys. The "Monk with a Big Head" was danced where there was space. The sound of drums and gongs mingled. Everywhere people crowded round to look." So there were age old lion dances and the "Big Head Show" which had been popular in the Song. "If there are no shows then the lanterns lose their sparkle, but if there are no dance troupes or drums and flutes then the flames die completely." (*Recollections of Tao An*). So obviously dance was indispensable at Lantern Festivals.

The Dew Book by Yao Lü of the Ming gives an account of the many kinds of folk dance he saw at Hongdong in Shanxi. These included the "Parasol Dance", in which small parasols were carried as the performers danced to the rhythm of the music, the "Huihui Dance" with dancing but no singing, and the "Flower Clapper Dance" where the dancers beat clappers as they danced as if their bodies were decked in flying flowers. In the early years after Liberation, a folk dance of the same kind existed in the Gansu area, large clappers being carried for the dance. There is a figure of a dancer carrying clappers on a Yuan mural in the Yulin caves at Anxi County, Gansu, so apparently such dance forms predated the Ming.

The "Rattan Shield Dance" which is common in Jiangxi, Zhejiang and Fujian evolved from the ancient "Axe and Shield Dance" and the Song "Tribal Shield Dance". There is a story that after the Ming national hero Qi Jiguang had defeated invading Japanese pirates, many of the demobilized troops settled along the coast in Zhejiang taking the "Rattan Shield Dance" from the army to the local people. Qi Jiguang took the drilling of his troops very seriously and was against "flowery methods" which were all form but no substance. However, he felt that "such 'flowery methods' cannot be avoided in 'Rattan Shield' when danced solo. In fact it is necessary to learn them. It contains feints, rolls and the like which are flowery methods". He also said, "All shields of rattan come from Fujian. Although they may be no defence against bullets, they can give cover against any stones, arrows, spears and swords. So they can replace armour and are very convenient in the muddy and rainy countryside of the South." As can be seen it was as an adaptation to the climate and geographic environment in the South that the "Rattan Shield Dance" came about. At the same time it also proves that legends that the dance originated from the fight against the Japanese led by Qi Jiguang in the Ming fit in with the historical facts. Other folk tales such as the "Songs and Dances for Heroes" also originated in the Ming.

At the Qing Lantern Festival or processions for idols, many kinds of folk arts were often brought together in composite performing units called "Shows at Religious Festivals" or in some places "Floral Circles". In form they were similar to the folk "Dance Troupes" of the Song. Included were such folk dances as the "Yangge", "Stilt Walking", "Lion Dance", "Thigh Drum", "Dry Boat", "Small Cart", "Bamboo Horse", "Monk with a Big Head", as well as martial arts like "Shaolin Boxing", "Five Tiger Sticks" and acrobatics "Pot Juggling", "Stone Lock Show" and "Harizontal Bar". There were also comic turns such as "Carrying the Box". The Qing painting of *A Religious Festival in Beijing* portrays all kinds of interesting performances in a clear and vivid way providing valuable figurative material for study of the subject (see figs.66-69).

Account of Seasonal Festivities in the Capital written by Pan Rongbi of the Qing records folk entertainments at the Lantern Festival in Beijing: "A variety of shows are put on at the Lantern Festival. Lanterns are made of colourful material.... There is Riding the Bamboo Horse, Catching Butterflies, skipping, hide-and-seek, dancing dragon lanterns, juggling sticks, tumbling and pole climbing as entertainment.... Performed at the Lantern Festival are the Monk with a Big Head and Yangge, the nine-act Yellow Flower Lantern, Exercise on the Horizontal Bar, Racing Bamboo Horses and the Taiping Spirit Drum."

Many of the folk dances from the Qing had already appeared in the Song as explained before. At this point let's discuss the

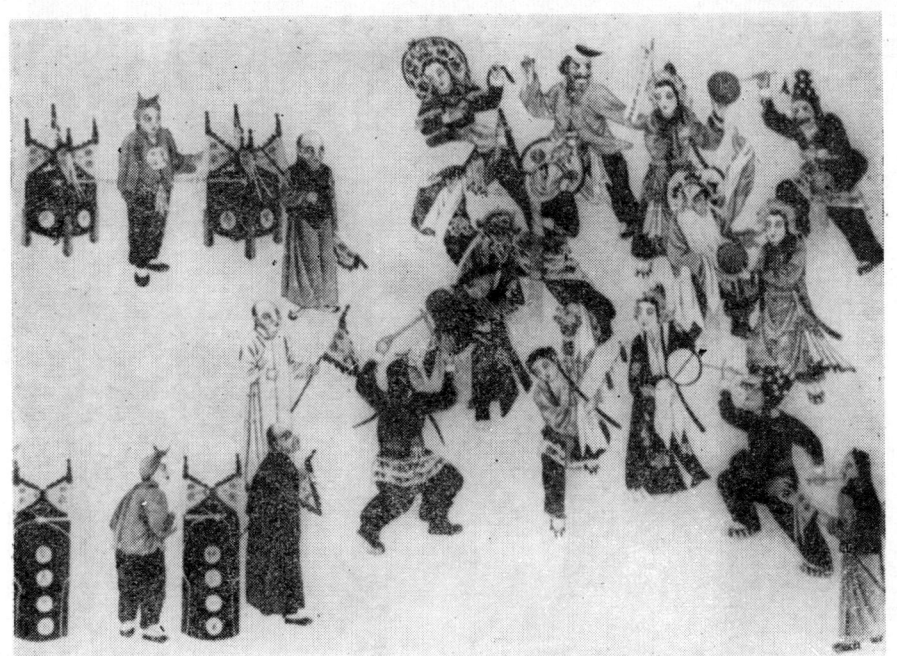
66. "Yangge" in the Qing painting *A Religious Festival in Beijing*.

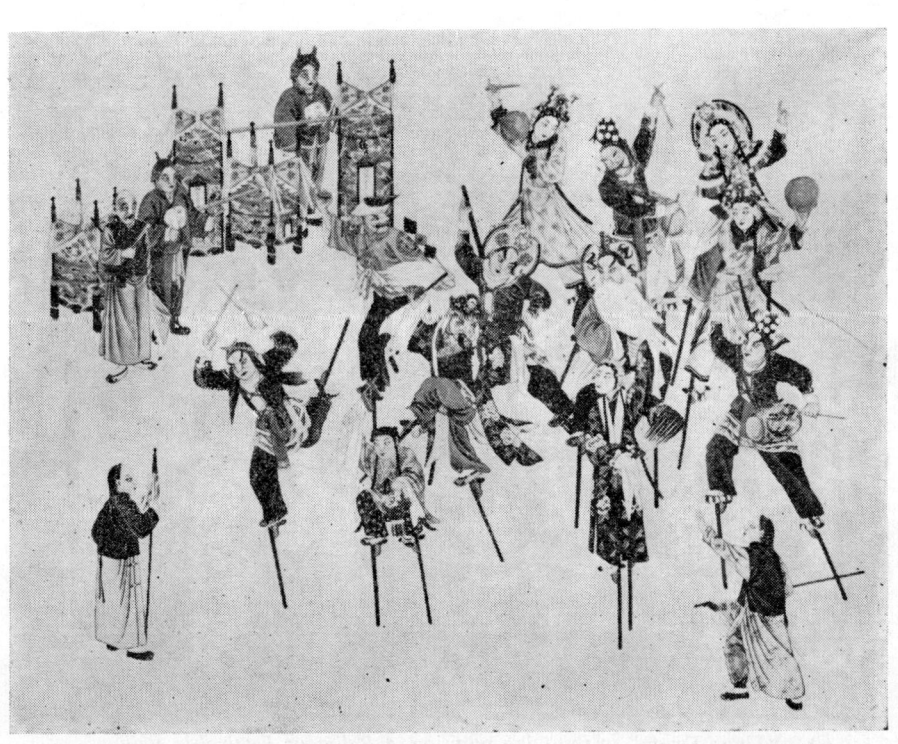
67. "Stilt Walking" in the Qing painting *A Religious Festival in Beijing*.

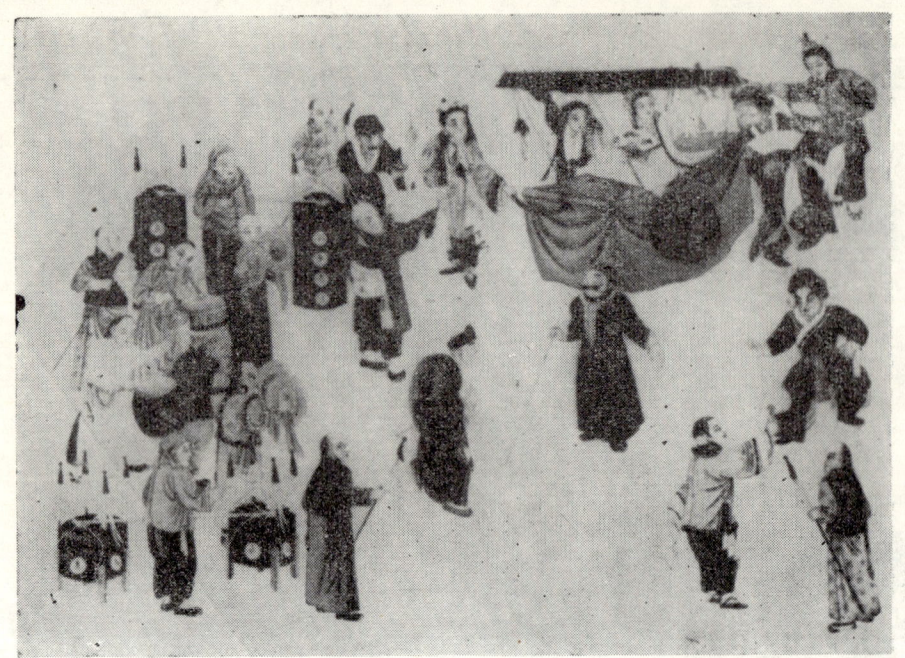

68. "Small Cart" in the Qing painting *A Religious Festival in Beijing*.

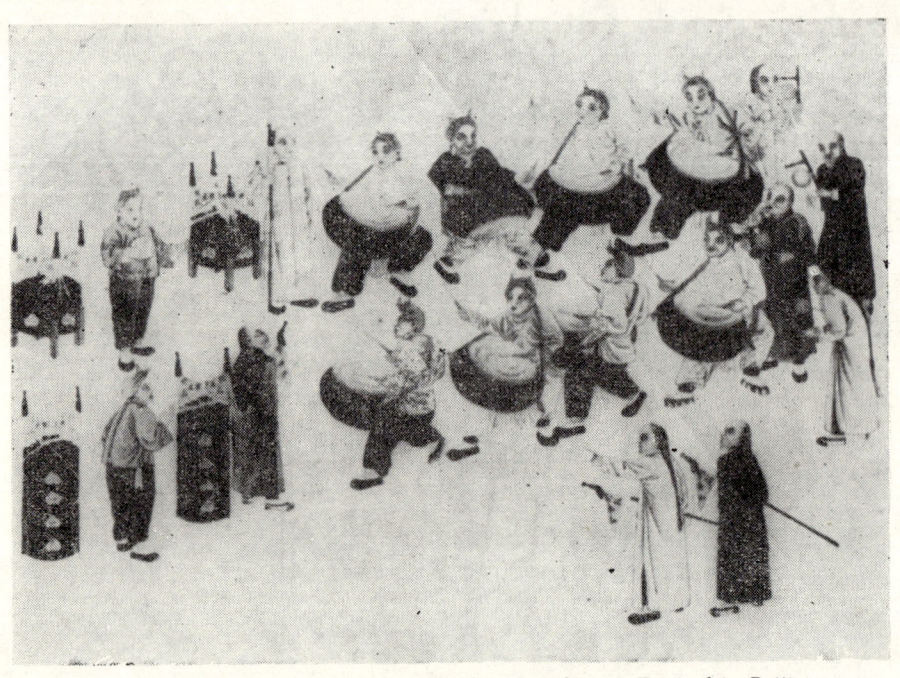

69. "Thigh Drum" in the Qing painting *A Religious Festival in Beijing*.

"Taiping Drum", "Yangge", and "Flower Drum Lantern" from Anhui in more detail.

Originally the Taiping Drum was a dance performed by shamans, hence the term "Taiping Spirit Drum". By the Qing, the instrument was already played as folk entertainment. *A Classified Collection of the Qing* says, "The New Year drum is bound by iron, with a bowl of wood joined onto the iron hoop. This is covered with skin which booms when hit. It is called the Taiping Drum and is played in the capital at the end of the year. Children enjoy it." This is the same as the popular Taiping Drum of today. He Er of the Qing describes the "Taiping Drum" dance of the time in the book *Miscellaneous Poems from Yantai*: "The iron hoop reverberates and the drum booms. Dancing becomes very popular as the year draws to a close. It seems as if there are Taiping drums everywhere; the sound of song on the streets is the same as that in the fields." In addition there is the "Poem about the Taiping Drum": "Covered in parchment light as silk-worm paper, it is carried in the left hand and hit with the right as an accompaniment for children. Its high and low rhythm sounds like the Dala drum, resounding through the alleys inside and outside the town." The *Poems from the Songfeng Pavilion*: "Boom boom sounds the Taiping Drum, children play at skipping in a bright, shiny circle. One child dances a second one sings, another child jumps into the shining ring. People crowd into the square from all around; throngs of fish and dragons celebrate New Year's Eve. Young girls climb bamboo poles 100 feet high. The beautiful kites fly in a clear breeze, beating their wings. Doors are unlocked tonight, and people walk the burnished moon-lit streets not returning home." Here there are descriptions of children skipping to the boom of the Taiping drum, the throngs of fish and dragons on the square (all kinds of dances imitating animals), the various shows on display and the crowds enjoying themselves in the moonlight who linger, reluctant to go home.

The "Yangge" originated in agricultural working life. The *Miscellaneous Poems for New Year* by Wu Xiqi of the Qing considers that the "Yangge" evolved from Song "Village Music". Since they both had the same kind of background it is quite probable they were of a common lineage. In his *Notes from Eastern Guangdong* the Qing author Li Diaoyuan writes, "In the countryside at springtime, women and children by the dozen would go to the fields to plant rice-seedlings. As the sound of a drum beaten by an old man, they competed together with group songs which lasted all day. It was called the Yangge." The Qing *Gazeteer for Huangzhou* printed in 1825 says: "In the spring, the peasants walk in the fields side by side. They use their feet as hoes to move the earth as they advance. A drum is beaten in rhythm at the side of the field. They go backwards or forwards quickly or slowly. It is partly as entertainment." This proves that when the rice seedlings were hoed, not only was a drum played and songs sung but they also advanced or retreated "dancing" either quickly or slowly to the rhythm of the music. These records fully demonstrate that music and dance in the "Yangge" arose from agricultural work.

The Yangge was not only popular in the countryside but in the towns as well then. "Small Yangge troupes performed in spring", and the congestion of people and carriages watching the "Yangge" was unbearable: "It was a furor with the hubs of wheels hitting against each other and people's shoulders rubbing together all the time" (from Ke Yu's *Folk Songs from the Capital*). Some people in troupes performing "Yangge Shows" wore costumes of a new design which aroused great interest. People flocked to see them: "When the Yangge first tried out clothes normally worn at home, the florid

Fengyang tunes were accompanied by drums. The hordes of onlookers could not be kept back but spilled over into the football field" (Yuan Qixu: *Folk Songs from the Capital*). The Yangge was mainly performed on street corners though sometimes at the theatre in between traditional operas. As Lu Youjia of the Qing writes in his *Folk Song from the Capital*: "The theatre takes on a new appearance in early spring, half of it is interspersed with Yangge as musical entertainment for the guests while they drink." Qing theatres doubled as drinking places. While plays or the "Yangge" were performed on stage the audience would watch and drink at the same time. The "Yangge" even reached the court. According to archives from the Shengping Bureau during the Qing Guangxu period: Ling Tong, Guang Fu and Ji Sheng were "Yangge instructors" at the Qing palace — proof that the Yangge was extremely popular then. The "Yangge Dance" has continued as the most widespread form of folk song and dance in China until the present day. Especially after the "Yangge" movement of 1942 at Yan'an, then the centre of the Chinese Revolution, this age-old dance was infused with fresh revolutionary content. It played a major role in the revolutionary struggle of the people and had a profound influence.

The many forms of "Flower Drum Lantern" are rich in local colour. In his *Folk Songs from the Capital* Ke Yu of the Qing says, "The florid Fengyang tunes were accompanied by drums", a reference to the "Fengyang Flower Drum" from Anhui which together with the "Flower Drum Lantern" was popular on both banks of the Huai River. The "Flower Drum Lantern" is said to have developed from the Ming "Playing the Red Lantern". According to old troupers it was in vogue in such areas as Fengtai and Huaiyuan during the Qing Guangxu period. There were small sites for performances by two or three people and big ones for larger numbers. The dance incorporated martial art movements making the dance idiom even more wild and vigorous thus depicting the bold, unbending spirit of the working people.

There are a large number of items in the "Flower Drum Lantern" praising the rebellious spirit of working people and denouncing the rapacious feudal code of ethics. According to what old artistes say "The Fourth Lord Sitting by Himself in the Sedan-Chair" made fun of landlords in a daring, trenchant style. It tells the story of two sedan-chair bearers, brave and resourceful peasants, who sauntered off quite nonchalantly after they had turfed out in mid-air the Fourth Lord, a landlord of great fastidiousness who found fault with everything. Such pieces also include sad melodies which attest to the terrible suffering inflicted on woman by feudal cash marriages: "He does not know me and I do not know him, whether scarred or pockmarked, deaf or dumb. I shall be married off for money. Mother, come and kill me!" Moreover, there were pieces singing of the genuine love of working people which at the same time condemned the cruel exploitation of the landlord class. "I clutch my love's hand in mine. It's not that I'm abandoning you. It's just that we cannot pay the rent so I'm going to be a slave girl in the landlord's house." Many of the lyrics in the "Flower Drum Lantern" voiced the true feelings of the working people.

The hard-working and wise inhabitants of China's vast territory created folk songs and dances of an incomparable beauty, some were in thanks for good harvests or in memory of a hero or portrayed the people's spirit of revolutionary struggle. Others exposed the violence and repulsiveness of the ruling class, ridiculing their greed and stupidity, or aired the terrible sufferings of the people or sought after a free and happy love life. In addition some dances depicted the cheerful outlook of working people. Whenever we probe into their origins or investigate their evolution and development, we discover that very many of these folk dances are several hundreds or even several thousands of years old. Even larger numbers originated in the Song, Yuan, Ming and Qing dynasties.

The feudal ruling class either altered folk dances for their own purposes or destroyed and banned them.

They were quite aware of the role of music and dancing arts in society. They would often use folk music and dance for their own political ends or for personal pleasure, sometimes performing them just as they were, at others rearranging the lyrics or adding "fine words". In some cases they also changed the dance's style or sentiments according to their own tastes in entertainment. Accounts of such examples have been given earlier on.

At this point we will discuss further the destruction and prohibition of folk dances by the feudal ruling class.

As early as the Tang Dynasty when the art of dancing was at its height the court had issued edicts banning folk song and dance. The Tang Emperor Xuanzong is famous in history for his love of song, dance and music-making — he even took a personal role in composing music and dance at court. In A.D. 751 he ordered the limit on the number of performers kept at private houses to be abolished. Yet it was the self same Xuanzong who issued command after command forbidding popular free form music (including folk music and dance). Among edicts promulgated in A.D. 714 was one which falsely accused folk music and dance and variety shows of being "harmful to decorum and government, but even worse they contravene the code of law and furthermore ought to be totally prohibited". In the tenth month of the same year there was another order "unclassified music is rife in the villages and really ought to be totally banned". "If anyone contravenes it", then the host who invited the artistes to perform and the village chief were to be flogged, the performers to be sentenced to hard labour.

In 1112 under the Song, Liu Huan, a Vice Minister at the Board of War, asked for "the vulgar music of actors and singing girls to be done away with" (that is popular free form music and variety shows). In 1113 the court again ordered that "vulgar songs from the past ... be completely forbidden, both the offenders and those listening should be tried for the crime". In this way, both the performers and their audience became criminals.

Coming as they did at the closing stages of feudal society there was an even greater stream of edicts for the prohibition and destruction of folk opera, music and dance in the Yuan, Ming and Qing dynasties, and we will only be giving bans on small folk song and dance shows and folk song and dance as examples. According to *Quotations from Banyan Village*, the "Ming Emperor Zhu Yuanzhang set up a tall tower in the street and ordered soldiers to stand watch on it. If they heard anyone secretly busking then the culprit would be immediately strung upside down from the tower and fed water for three days when they would die".

From 1671 onwards during the Qing, decrees were issued on numerous occasions banning Yangge singing processions. Anyone who hired Yangge artistes to give performances was to be punished with a flogging. The *Miscellaneous Transcripts of Recent Proclamations* contains the following account of a decree published in Jiangsu in 1718 banning the "Yangge" and "Dragon Lantern". "At New Year Lantern Festivals the Yangge is sung and tricks performed ... puppets dance, dragon lanterns are played.... An immediate investigation is called for so the districts can be pacified." In 1835 there was an edict banning stilt performances in addition to which in 1850 there was the affair of Liu Shi, a Yangge artiste, who was arrested and persecuted. In March 1867, the former provincial governor of Jiangsu had a stone tablet erected forbidding performances of the Flower Drum and Wuxi rhymed storytelling at teahouses in Yuanmiaoguan. *The Record of Proclamations* contains an edict strictly forbidding performances of Tea Picking: "Since the New Year, performances of Tea Picking have continued every night. From now on ... stages should no longer be put up ... nor charges collected for performances of Tea Picking. The name of anyone not complying with this prohibitions notice should be immediately furnished to the district authorities by the local leader or others. Those in charge of the performers and fathers or brothers who have allowed their sons to sing must all be flogged without mercy." What a terrible ban! Even the fathers and brothers of the actors were to be punished with beatings as well. Since they were sung over successive nights these shows were of course very popular. There are also accounts in the *Notes on the Seasons at Yanjing* of local officials prohibiting "shows at religious festivals". Such harsh bans on folk arts by the feudal ruling class met with strong resistance on the part of ordinary people. According to an account in *Memoranda from Hunan and Hubei*, some government officials in the Qing issued official notices prohibiting folk "shows at religious festivals" but the local people ignored it and continued making enthusiastic preparations for a procession with performances of a variety of folk arts. Just as they were about to set out, the government office published yet another prohibition order. Everybody begged them to cancel it but the county government would not do so. Popular feeling ran high. The main hall of the local officials was torn down, set fire to and burnt to the ground. These was no stopping them and only after the local authorities had been forced to adopt conciliatory measures did the crowds disperse. However, subsequently the authorities seized the two leaders, Wang and Cao, and had them killed. Why did the feudal ruling class hate folk dance so much that they destroyed and banned it out of hand? It was because of their fear of the people "assembling to rebel" and their fear of the people unmasking them and rising in revolt. However, over thousands of years the populace had experienced much suffering and unrest due to war. Folk dance had been banned many times yet it had continued to be handed down from generation to generation to be preserved right up until before Liberation — though there were some folk dances which had died out or were on the verge of doing so. After Liberation, especially in the fifties and early sixties, the folk dances of each ethnic group blossomed in all their glory under the protective care of the Party. Through being collected, arranged, worked on and improved, many folk dances have formed a dance art beloved by people in China as well as the rest of the world.

CHAPTER NINE

Dances of the National Minorities

China is a unified, multi-national state. Besides the Han who make up over 90 per cent of the population, there are more than 50 national minorities. The people of China have shared the same land for a long period of time. Through good times and bad they have been brought together through the influence they have had on each other and created in common the great cultural tradition of the Chinese people. A fine dance tradition is included therein. Each national minority's dance has its own long history and distinctive style. Due to limits on the material we could manage, only a rough introduction based on the historical data presented here is possible.

Before Liberation, there was a vast imbalance in the social development of different national minority areas due to the reactionary rule of the exploiting class and various historical reasons. Some were in the state of Feudal Society while others at that of Slave Society. There were even some which still retained vestiges of the Primitive Commune. Only a few of them had their own script, some had a rudimentary writing system, the majority lacked any at all. Often the history of the growth of each nationality's dances depended on an oral tradition handed down over the years. Moreover Han historical documents contain only a few fragmentary records.

The work, life, love and customs of national minorities are closely bound up with their dance. Large group dances are common and have retained their distinctive national traits. They are in a simple, wholesome style which breathes with life.

The Mongol, Tibetan, Uygur, Miao, Korean, Yao, Dai and other nationalities have always been renowned for their song and dance skills. Their dancing art holds an important place in the history of Chinese dance.

As long ago as the Xia Dynasty when Shaokang came to the throne (in about the 21st century B.C.) there were "Tribal guests from the borders who presented their songs and dances". Which nation the "tribal guests" refers to can no longer be verified but it is probable that song and dance exchange between nationalities did in fact occur.

The "Music from Distant Regions" set up by the Zhou court was for national minority song and dance from all areas. There were set performances for specific occasions. This method was followed by the feudal ruling classes down through the ages with "Music from Distant Regions" being set up at the palace. It was to vaunt their own strength that they acted in this way. Political motives were involved. Moreover the performance of such national minority pieces at court did, objectively speaking, play a role in the dissemination and exchange of music and dance from each nation.

After Zhang Qian toured the Western Regions during the Han, music and dance from there and other places were conveyed to central China. According to *Miscellaneous Records of the Western Capital*, "Khotan Music" already formed part of the repertoire for court festivals in the early Han. On leaving the palace, Jia Peilan, servant to the Han Emperor Gaozu's favourite concubine Lady Qi, talked of entertainments there: "On the seventh day of the seventh month, Khotan music is performed by the Baizi Pool." Ancient Khotan corresponds to present day Hotan County in Xinjiang. Since days of old it has been a fertile area for folk song and dance. In the *Record of the Western Regions in the Great Tang*, Xuanzang who lived then says, "The Kingdom of Kustana (i.e. Khotan) ... is a country where music is revered, and the people are fond of singing and dancing." During the Han "Khotan Music" Spread in the Central Plains area and was much liked by the Han people though, as mentioned before, the Bayu Dance of the Cong national minority from the Southwest had an even greater influence then.

The two Jin and Southern and Northern Dynasties were periods when there was a great deal of exchange of national minority music and dance, periods when the various nationalities were brought together through the influence they had on each other.

Tang music and dance absorbed the strong points from such pieces as well as those from abroad in great quantities and thus a new form of national music and dance was created. Each of the peoples in China made their own due contribution to this great development in ancient dancing arts.

The "Dance to Foreign Music" performed at Song "Wazi", the "Tartar Dance" put on at folk festivals and the "Mulberry Branch Dance" which was popular in the Tang and continued on into the Song all testify to the spread of national minority music and dance in the area of the Han people.

With the rise of traditional opera after the Song and Yuan, Han and national minority dances were seldom performed as separate art forms. Consequently there was a decline in systematic records in history books. The circumstances surrounding the development of national minority dance can be glimpsed here and there in notes and jottings. Although not systematic they are factual, vivid and reliable as their authors would often only write something down once they had seen it themselves. We will now give a brief description of some of the historical background to several national minority dances.

The Uygurs who mostly live in Xinjiang have enjoyed a long history. The area around Xinjiang used to be known as the "Western Regions" in ancient times. Contacts between China proper and the "Western Regions" were strengthened after Zhan Qian toured the area in 139 B.C. As early as 60 B.C., the Han Dynasty established a "Garrison in the Western Regions" and in the Tang a "Garrison at Anxi" and a "Garrison at Beiting" were also set up. From then on each dynasty established administrative machinery in Xinjiang. In the Han and Tang, especially the Tang, the Central Plains were inundated with music and dance from Xinjiang. They were very popular with the Han people living there and had quite an influence.

The "Twelve Mukamu" are large song and dance pieces popular amongst the Uygurs. Their contents are varied including songs of recitation, folk narrative singing suites, series of dances and musical improvisations — more than 340 pieces in all which have been handed down for many centuries. While in Xinjiang in 1963 members of the Chinese Musical Research Institute collected the *Brief History of Artistes* written in 1854 by Maola Yisimutula. It gives brief biographies of 17 artists and mentions how popular the "Mukamu" they wrote were. Aibunaisier Falabi who composed the famous piece "Yuzihaer Mukamu" is an example. Maiwulana Yili wrote the celebrated "Iraq and Gobi Mukamu" after traversing Iraq and the Gobi. Abudurehemai Jiami who died in 1481 wrote two sections of the "Aijiemu" Mukamu. The "Nawayi Mukamu" by Yilixier Nawayi was known far and wide, its author died in 1489. Xiayehe Shapayi knew all there was to know about Mukamu and died in 1452. Maimaiti Kuxitigeer composed famous Mukamu songs like the "Qiahaerzenaifu" and died in 1482. As can be seen from the above accounts, this kind of large song and dance piece, the "Mukamu", was at the least over 500 years old. Moreover the "Survey of Uygur Literature and Arts" believes the "Twelve Mukamu" are more than 1,300 years old.

There are many other fine Uygur folk dances of long-standing such as the "Sainaimu". The many graceful dancing poses in this extremely widespread group dance endow it with a beautiful lyricism. Investigations show that during the course of their formation the "Twelve Mukamu" incorporated the Sainaimu which had already been popular for many years. Obviously then it must have been even older.

The time honoured "Daolang Mukamu" which circulates in the southern part of Xinjiang, has its own unique style. "Daolang" meant "Tulan" in ancient Uygur (i.e. "crowd"). Long, long ago people in the areas bordering the Tarim Desert took part in communal labour so they were called "Daolang" people. This is also said to have been the general term for the inhabitants of the Tarim River. The "Daolang Mukamu" has a set structural form. The first section consists of a loosely rhythmed solo sung in sonorous tones. "Qieketeman", the second part, has a slow, steady beat. Everybody sings in unison as the dancers invite each other to dance in pairs. "Sainaimu" comes next, a moderately paced dance piece in which a couple dance together twisting as they move along. The fourth piece the "Kenaikesi" is an exuberant number with a clear rhythm. Everybody dances in a circle. The fifth section, "Sailiman", is an allegro. They circle round twisting and wheeling wildly and end up spinning rapidly on the spot. The entire dance thus culminates in a climax. Other works such as the stirring "Sama Dance" or the beautiful "Hand Drum Dance" with its many dancing postures have all been in existence for a long time.

The Mongols are a nationality from the northern regions of China formed from many tribes over a long period of historical development. Only when Genghis Khan unified the tribes in the area of Mongolia in the 13th century did they become generally known as the "Mongols".

Most Mongolian dances are strong and vigorous yet at the same time some are beautifully evocative.

The "Dance of the Sixteen Demons" at the Yuan* court was probably a religious dance with distinctive Mongolian features. The *History of the Yuan Dynasty* contains the following description, "A slow dance performed by 16 girls from the Court.... It is called the Sixteen Demons. Their hair hangs in braids from their heads and they wear Buddhist mitres of ivory. Their bodies draped in tassels they have long and short skirts in crimson silk and gold with gold-speckled jackets. They wear stoles, sacred garments with closed sleeves and beribboned shoes and stockings. They each carry a Buddhist prayer instrument, and one of them plays on a bell with a baton." Performances were given when "Buddhist services" were held at the palace. Ye Shijie of the late Yuan and early Ming records that, "In the Yuan there was the Dance of the Sixteen Demons. Sixteen beautiful women adorned with pearls and tassels danced to the image of

---
*The Yuan Dynasty was founded by the Mongols and lasted from 1271-1368.

the Bodhisattva." Later on this dance spread amongst the people too. The ruling class issued an edict banning it which went, "Stop singing the Sixteen Demons, stop performing it in poetic dramas, stop playing it.... If there are any infringements the culprits must be punished." It was due to the very fact that the dance had become popular that it incurred a ban.

After Genghis Khan united the country, Mongolian music and dance, such as the "Daola" which was handed down from the Yuan right up until the Qing, spread to the Central Plains. *Old Stories from Previous Dynasties* says that "The Daola has brought with it a new kind of work; the dance with bowl lanterns is even lighter. Zithers and lutes play together accompanied by brass instruments." A note in the original went, "In the Yuan there was the Daola Show, the name for a song.... They also danced with bowl lanterns on their heads." The music had a distinctive Mongolian style with the dancers carrying lanterns on their heads for the dance.

Lu Ciyun describes how the "Daola" was performed, the music started up and "the dancers in dignified dancing poses each carry a bowl on their heads, and on the top is a lighted lamp. Speckled bamboo is carried inside the mouth to mark the rhythm being pleasant to listen to". Then he tells how the music played faster and faster as the dancers wheeled round like swirling snow. It was a wonderful performance which greatly impressed the audience. This piece has many points of similarity with the "Lantern Dance" and "Bowl Dance". Both are Mongolian dances which have been handed down until the present day so they can be said to be in the same tradition. The Mongolian people are adept at song and dance and have created a rich music and dance tradition.

The ancestors of the Tibetans were the "Qiang", known as the "Tufan" in the Tang. The Han and Tibetan peoples have always had a close relationship. In A.D. 641, the Tang princess Wencheng was married to a Tibetan king called Songzanganbu. In A.D. 710 another princess, Jincheng, was married to King Chidezuzan. The story of these two princesses going to Tibet still circulates widely amongst the Tibetan people. There is also a Tibetan play about Princess Wencheng going there. In A.D. 823 a stone tablet was erected to the alliance between the Tang and Tufan (Tibetan) marking the friendly relations between the two peoples. It remains preserved to this very day in front of the Jokhan Monastery at Lhasa.

There are two late Tang murals in Cavern No. 156 at Dunhuang, the *Picture of Zhang Yichao Setting Out* (see fig. 70) and that of his wife *Picture of Madame Songguo Setting Out* (see fig. 71). Among the imposing ranks of departing troops are some artists in the guard of honour who are also travelling with them. Eight male dancers dance opposite each other in two rows. The stance and dress are very similar to present day Tibetan dances. Their arms are held out obliguely while they seem to be stamping with their feet. Four women dancers are in a square formation. They wear Han national dress — skirts and jackets, sashes draped over their shoulders and wavy cloud patterned shoes. Their dancing poses are quite like traditional Tibetan song and dance forms — poses often used in the "Xianzi" dance. Some people think it is the Tang "Xiliang Arts". Judging from the style of the dancing postures it includes quite a number of features typical of Tibetan dance. The area of Dunhuang in the Gansu Corridor was originally a gateway for communications between the main area of China and the Western Regions. Since it was a place inhabited by people of various nationalities there would have been frequent cultural contacts. Zhang Yichao was a Military Governor sent to

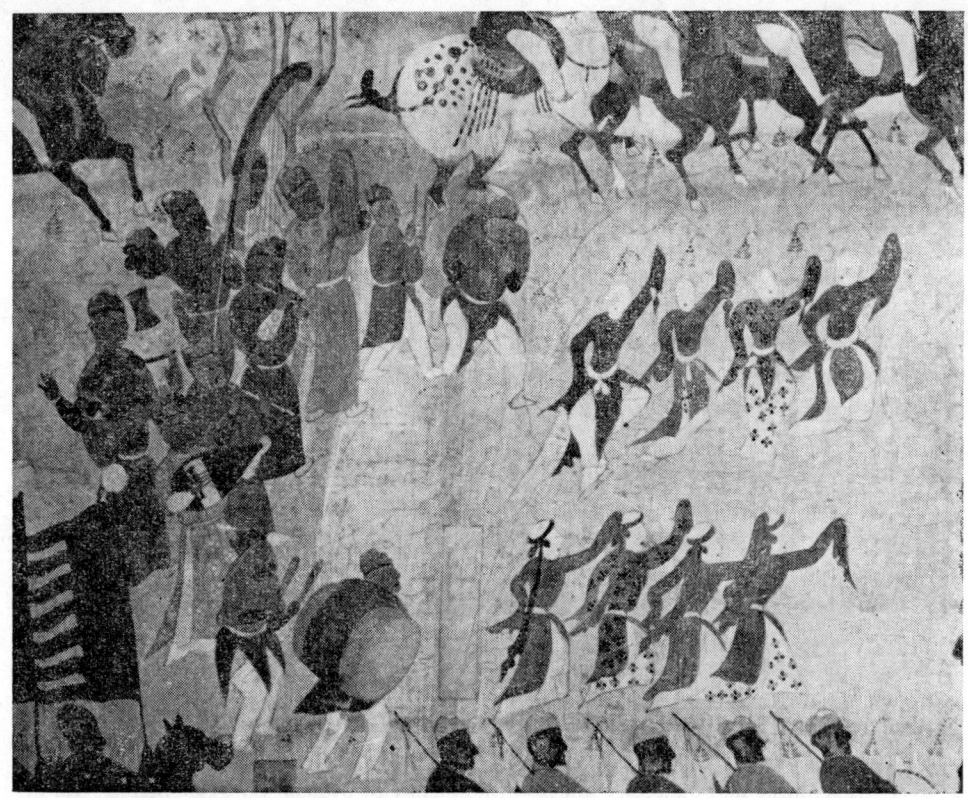
70. The music and dance section from the *Picture of Zhang Yichao Setting Out* on a Tang mural at Dunhuang from Cavern No. 156 at the Mogao Caves.

garrison the region. His troops included many different nationalities so there would certainly have been national minority musicians and dancers amongst the camp performers in his army.

The Tibetan people are skilled at song and dance. Many of their folk dances date back a long way.

The "Zhuo" — the "Guozhuang Dance" — is said to be already some 500 or 600 years old. One of Dege's lyrics to the "Guozhuang" goes, "The Dalai Lama from Rear Tibet". Only the first and second Dalai Lamas lived there. Calculating from the time of the first Dalai Lame, that would be more than 500 years ago.

"Guozhuang Dance" movements can be roughly divided into two types — those which are lingering and graceful with a slow rhythm and those with a rapid tempo and frenetic actions. Many of the dance movements are supposed to be imitations of animal forms such as the "Fierce Tiger Descends the Mountain", "Soaring of the Mighty Eagle", "Peacocks Spread Their Feathers" and "Gambolling of Wild Animals". These relate to the hunting life of people in the region. This is reflected in some of the lyrics too which also contain expressions of love or sing the praises of their native places.

Later on the "Guozhuang Dance", the creation of ordinary people, was tampered with for use by the ruling class of slave owners. For example performances of the "Great Guozhuang" were restricted to set sacrificial ceremonies, commoners (the serfs) could not dance it when they liked. A line in the lyrics to the "Guozhuang" goes, "The

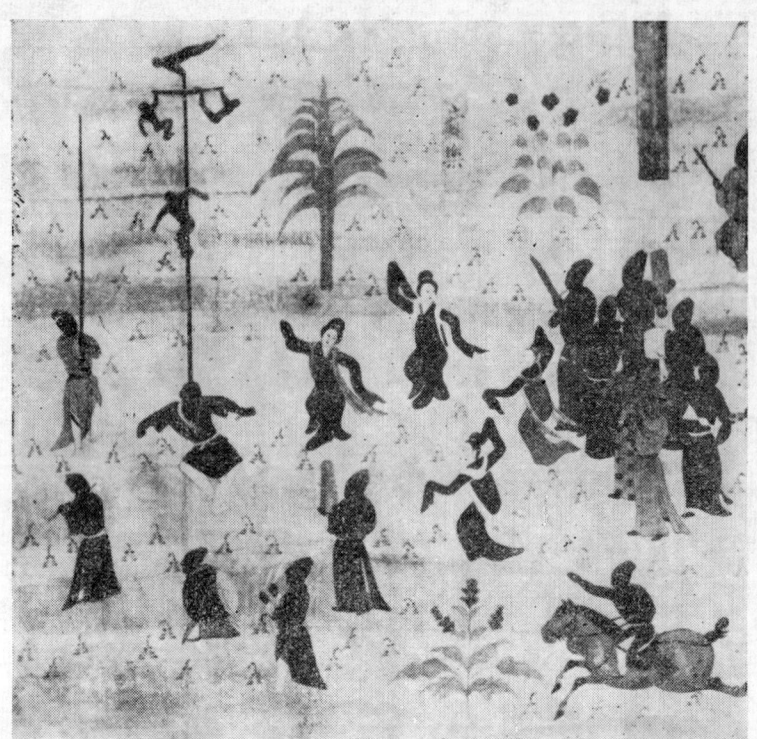

71. The music and dance section from the *Picture of Madam Songguo Setting Out* on a Tang mural at Dunhuang from Cavern No. 156 at the Mogao Caves.

Guozhuang must be danced well so must the Peacock Eating Grapes. Good dances cannot be danced as you will, but only after the lamas have spun their prayer wheels.... The Guozhuang must be danced well and so must the Spirit Eagle of the Universe. Good dances cannot be danced as you will, but only when the headmen organize them".

A story circulating in the Aba region tells of a slave who used dance in his struggle with a headman. Once upon a time in the Maer area lived a terribly brutal headman. The people hated him through and through, so they composed a "Guozhuang Dance" called "Yibu Gongjian" (i.e., "Bow and Arrow Dance"). An arrow was hidden in the sleeve of the lead dancer who shot the headman dead while performing for him.

The *Illustrated Record of Garrisons in Tibet* printed in the Qing says the Tibetans habitually danced the "Guozhuang" pieces. More than 10 women wearing hats ringed with white material and clothed in colourful garments stood hand in hand in a circle. "Lifting their feet, they sing and dance in a ring." This kind of "Guozhuang Dance" danced by women included fairly big leaps as well as twisting movements.

A work for officials in the Qing to study geography the *Maps of Tribute to the Imperial Qing* says that: "The Zagu were originally a Tibetan tribe in the Tang. When a boy and girl fell in love they sang and danced hand in hand. It was called the 'Guozhuang' ", a form of Guozhuang dance in which men and women danced together much the same as the modern day version still widespread among the Tibetans.

There are other time-honoured Tibetan songs and dances such as the "Xie" — the

"Xianzi Dance". A man playing a Xianzi, a two-stringed fiddle, leads the dance at the front. He is followed by a crowd of people singing and dancing in a circle. They gently toss their long sleeves to the sweet, lingering melody in soft, graceful dancing poses. For the "Duixie" — in Han usage it would be known as a "Tap Dance" — the feet are used in kicking, treading, leaping, dancing, stamping and brushing movements to convey a variety of clear-cut, complicated rhythms through the dancing. It has a cheery spirit and strong, forceful dancing poses. There is also the "Reba Dance", a composite performance in which bell and drum dances, acrobatics, joke-telling and all kinds of folk dances are included. Lively and uninhibited in form, it is mostly performed as a living by folk "Reba" artists. Investigations by theatre personnel since Liberation show that these dances were already quite popular in the Qing.

The forerunners of the Yao nationality were known in Qin and Han times as the "Wuyi Barbarians of Changsha" (a derogatory term for national minorities in feudal history books). In the Sui and Tang they were called the "Moyao" and there are a fair number of records to do with the Yao people from the Song Dynasty. Zhou Qufei who lived then was once a government official at Guilin in Guangxi. On returning to his home in the east he wrote a book called *Answers About the Other Side of the Mountains* in response to questions from his guests. In it is noted the way of life of several national minorities he himself had seen. When mentioning the homage paid to the "Great King Dubei" by the Yao in the 10th month every year, he writes, "Men and women each in groups, danced side by side. It was called the Tayao. When a boy and girl fell in love with each other, the man would shout giving a great leap, enter the women's group and carry his love back off home. They then became man and wife."

It's a lively description of an ancient Yao custom whereby when group dances were held at festivals, young people would choose their own boy or girl friends as they danced, arranging their own marriage contracts. An account of the custom of "Men and women getting together for singing and dancing" amongst Yao living in the areas of Chenzhou and Yuanzhou in Hunan is also given in *Notes from the Laoxue Convent* by Lu You of the Song.

Another Song writer, Shen Liao, says in his "Dancing and Wheeling Pieces" that "To east and west of the Xiang River they dance and wheel. There are blue smoke, white mist and giant trees. During the festival drink is free. The muse of music holds forth on the long waist drums. Girls in bangles and plain silk, laugh happily as they chase boys — the spirits are in control. The following spring they will bring wine and oxen to visit the parents". Performing the "Dance of the Long Drum" in homage to the gods and choosing one's own sweetheart are ancient Yao customs. The poem gives a clear description of how folk dancing at Yao festivals in the Song actually was.

There are similar accounts in the *Book of Merits and Failings of the Various Kingdoms in the Empire* by Gu Yanwu who lived during the Ming: "People from Hunan hold processions in honour of Pan Gu* . . . now known under a different name as it is taboo. On the day of the procession, they use wooden drums larger than a peck measure in diameter, empty in the middle and large at both ends. The one four feet in length is called the long drum. The other of two feet the short drum. . . . A sorcerer dances with a long drum round his body, two other people carrying short drums dance facing each other." This is an even more lucid and factual description of the Yao

---

* According to Chinese myth Pan Gu was creator of the Universe.

"Long Drum Dance". To this day there are both large and small types of Yao long drum. Their shape remains as it was, large at either end and narrow in the middle. It is held by its waist and hit throughout the dance.

Kuang Lu of the Ming left his home town as he had opposed the local officials. He went to live for a fairly long time in the national minority area of Guangxi and wrote a book, the *Chi Ya*. It is an account of the customs and habits as well as song and dance activities of the many national minorities living there. Included are descriptions of Yao customs: the paying of homage to Pan Gu and music-making, singing and dancing by both sexes. Mention is also made of their "worship of the Great King Dubei. In a dance known as the Tayao, men and women dance side by side. When they fall in love with each other they leap and dance and leave with the girl being carried." Almost exactly the same as the accounts from the Song.

In *Notes from the West of Guangdong* edited by Zhang Xianghe of the Qing it says, "Of Yao customs the best is their singing and dancing." Men and women, wearing beautifully coloured costumes, sang and danced deep in the lush bamboo forests.

There are depictions of each national minority in *Scenic Views of the Country* printed during the Qing. One section consists of illustrations of dance poses including pictures of Yao dancing (see fig. 72). Both men and women have their hair in buns and wear earrings. The women are clad in colourful skirts with long sashes draped across their bodies. They raise their hands and tramp their feet dancing as the men follow behind. An explanation identifies them as being several national minorities from Libo County in Guizhou including the Dong and Yao. To celebrate New Year they had to pay homage to Pan Gu. "The men and women dance side by side when they fall in love the men carry the women off home and are then married."

The Qing *Gazette of the Lianshan Subprefecture for Pacifying the Yao* remarks that

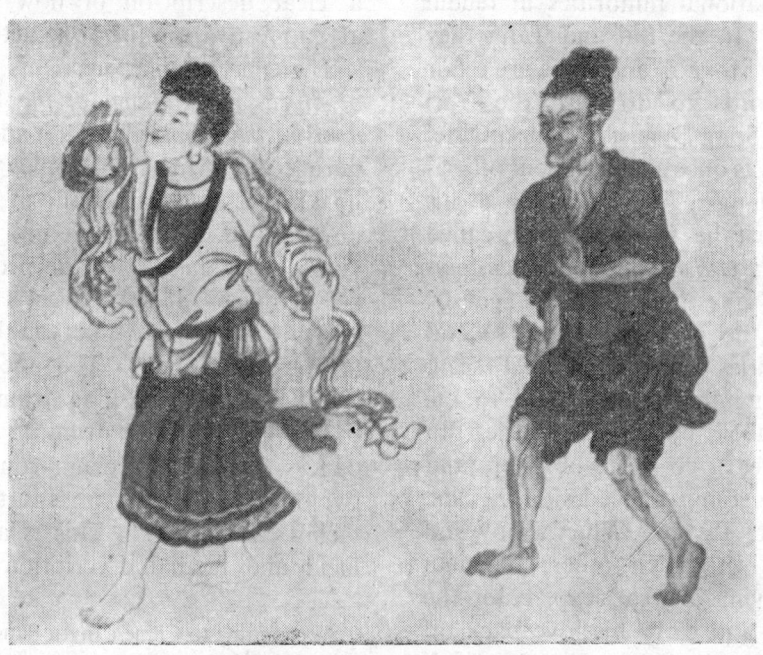

72. A Yao dance in the Qing.

the Yao long drum "is made of wood. Though both ends are of the same diameter, the middle is slim like a waist." It also says that they hit the drum with their hands as they danced.

The above accounts prove that the Yao in Guangxi, Hunan and Guangdong shared the same customs which remained virtually unchanged for the 700 or 800 years from the Song and Yuan till the Ming and Qing. The "Long Drum Dance" has a long history for there were already reliable reports in the Song so it must have been even earlier in origin. It has continued down to the present day as the main form of dance most enjoyed by Yao people. By and large labouring work such as the building of houses or construction of long drums is depicted. There is the "Civilian Long Drum" which has beautiful dancing poses whereas the "Military Long Drum" consists of wild and vigorous movements. Since Liberation an arrangement called the "Long Drum Dance of the Yao" has been made based on Yao folk dances.

The history of the Miao is a long one. Some people believe that the "Three Miao" of legend in Primitive Society were actually their forebears. During Qin and Han times, feudal history books derogatorily termed them "Savages of the Five Streams" or "Wuyi Barbarians". Though there are records of the Miao in the Tang and Song the word was sometimes used as a general term for national minorities in the south.

The *Chi Ya* states that: "The Miao are themselves a type, the women ... can dance like mynahs." The word "Mynah Dance" first occurs in the Jin Dynasty. At a banquet Xie Shang performed this dance, "bending and raising his head in the middle, oblivious of the audience." It is difficult to ascertain whether the "Mynah Dance" of Miao in Guangdong during the Ming was the same as that danced by Xie Shang in the Jin or not. However, they were both probably dances which imitated bird movements. Such mimicry of animals in dance dates back a long way. In 1952 we listened to the following story told us by an elderly Miao inhabitant from Fuxing township, a remote mountain district in the Danzhai Miao Autonomous County in Guizhou. Long, long ago there was a young Miao man who went hunting in the mountains and brought back a gorgeous mynah bird as catch. He asked his wife to wear a headdress and costume in imitation of the bird's appearance. He then went on to start performing this kind of bird dance with her. The costumes of the Miao women in this mountainous area differ from those in other places. They tie their hair in high buns, have tight fitting clothes and trousers and wear short flounced skirts with pleats. Their aprons are in two parts, short in front and long behind. From the back of the waist trail beautifully coloured ribbons of differing lengths. When they perform the Reed Pipe Dance, their headdresses dip and shake as the coloured ribbons on their skirts flash to and fro. With palms tilted upwards slightly they hold their arms a little apart and wave them to and fro for all the world like a beautiful mynah. Though we do not know exactly the form the "Mynah Bird Dance" took as performed by Miao in Guangdong during the Ming we *do* know there is a legend that Miao dance originated from imitations of bird behaviour.

The Miao "Reed Pipe Dance" has a long history. It is the most widespread and common of dances amongst the Miao. A man playing a reed pipe usually leads followed behind by women dancing to the music. An account in the *Imperial Compendium* says that amongst Miao in Yunnan "A man playing a reed pipe leads, men and women with arms linked dance round and round for pleasure." The illustration to the "Reed Pipe Dance" (see fig. 73) in the *Beautiful Sights from All over the Country* depicts a

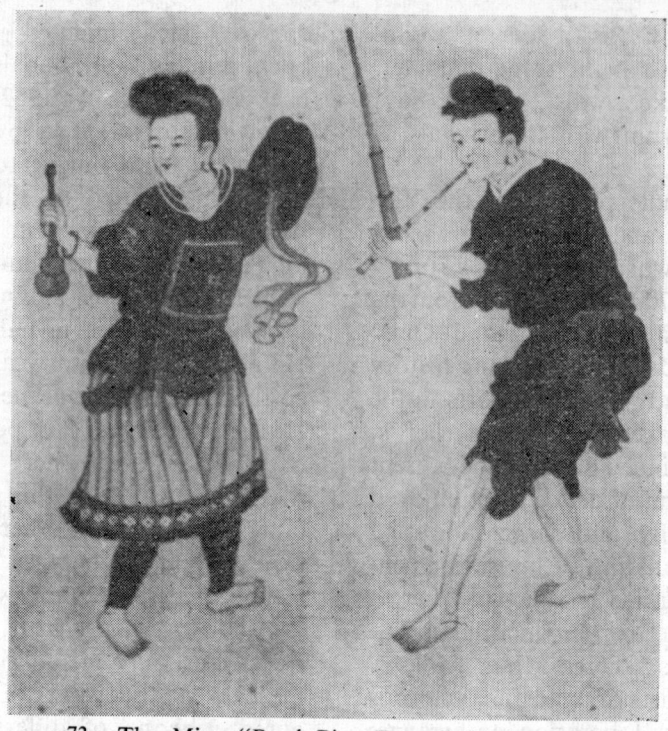
73. The Miao "Reed Pipe Dance" in the Qing.

Miao youth playing a reed pipe as he dances. A woman in a tall bun and wearing a coloured skirt and costume carries a sash in her left hand and shakes a bell in her right hand as she dances. The note to the picture reads: A custom of the Miao: "Every year in the first month of spring, a flat spot called a moon arena is chosen. A man plays a reed pipe and a woman a bell. They circle singing and dancing. It is called the Moon Dance." This custom has remained popular even after Liberation in Miao areas. The shape of the pipe is much the same as that in the Qing, only there is not just one man playing but many. When the women dance they do not carry sashes or bells but generally dance empty-handed.

The Zhuang are the most populous of the national minorities in China. The Huashan Cliff Murals are important historical data telling us about the life of their ancestors (the Zhuang Autonomous Region Museum in Guangxi dates them from the Warring States Period). They are mostly spread along cliffs on both banks of the Mingjiang and Zuojiang Rivers in the southwest of the Zhuang Autonomous Region in Guangxi. The biggest murals with the largest number of figures are at Huashan in Ningming County from which they get their name. Scenes of large gatherings and happy crowds singing and dancing are portrayed: the people stand in lines with hands held high and knees bent. Some are standing on one leg with the other "drawn back" as if they are dancing forwards together in a group. There are also a lot of figures with arms held up in the "riding crouched down" pose. Pictured here and there among the crowds are bronze drums with sun patterns and circular instruments like gongs. The fact that they appear makes it clear that the crowds of people neatly lined up in different postures are scenes from a mass song and dance (see fig. 74). According to what dance personnel there say, these dancing poses from the

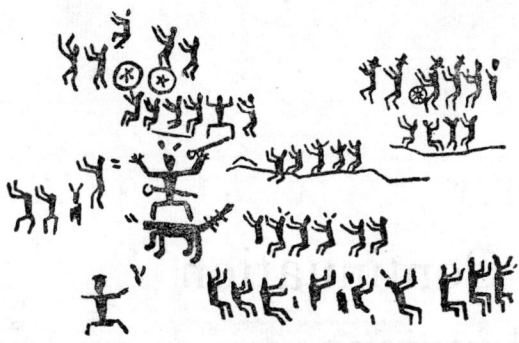

74. Copy of part of the Huashan cliff murals in Guangxi.

Huashan murals have been preserved till the present day in ancient Zhuang folk dances such as the "Shigong Dance". The bronze drum was the main Zhuang musical instrument in times gone by and had extremely beautiful line decorations. On some there are carvings of dancing figures like the one unearthed at a Western Han tomb at Luopo Bay in Guixian County, Guangxi. Twenty dancers wearing feather headdresses are carved on the waist of the drum. They are half-naked on top and wear skirts which are short in the front and long at the back. Their hands and arms are adorned with hanging ornaments (see fig. 75).

Besides these there are many other national minority folk dances with a long history such as the Korean "Long Drum Dance" and "Country Music Dance", the "Axi Moon Dance" of the Yi people, the Dai "Peacock Dance" the Li people's "Money Bell and Double Sword Dance", the Zhuang "Carrying Pole Dance" and the Gaoshan nationality's "Pestle Dance".

The foundations of the national minority dance tradition in China are extremely solid. Before Liberation the national minorities were subject to all kinds of oppression but even under such extreme circumstances they carried on their own cultural and art traditions. Although the rate of development was extremely slow they did after all keep them going. The main reason was that the dances sprang from the life of the people and had deep roots therein. Through song and dance they sang of their history, educated the younger generation, praised their native places and gave expression to feelings of love. Song and dance became an indispensable part in the lives of the people of the national minorities.

After Liberation, led by the Chinese Communist Party, national minorities throughout the country smashed the fetters of slavery and took the socialist road. There were unprecedented improvements in their dances, just as the late Mao Zedong describes in a line from a poem:

Now the cock has crowed and all under heaven is bright,
Here is music from all our peoples, from Khotan too.

People from the national minorities in China feted victory at Liberation in song and dance. The age-old dancing arts of the various nationalities blossomed in their full glory in the new China as well as on the international stage. Such achievements have already far outstripped those of the golden age for dance in ancient China — the Tang Dynasty.

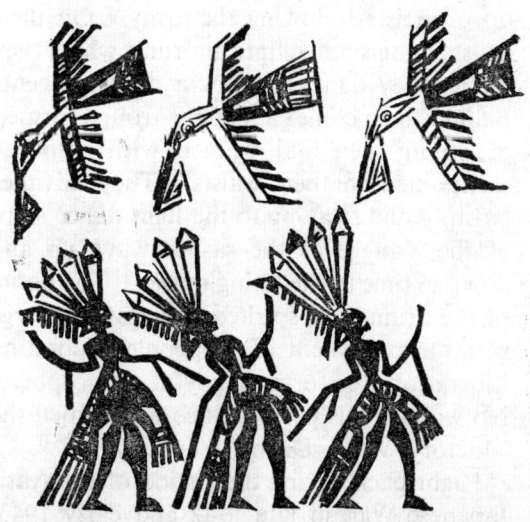

75. Copy of part of a design on a bronze drum from the Western Han.

APPENDIX
Thirty Years of Continuation and Development

During the late forties in the wake of the Chinese People's Liberation Army, the sound of drums and Yangge songs resounded the length and breadth of the land. It was the first time for years that the newly liberated populace in the cities, towns and countryside could again enjoy traditional dance. The liberation of the people brought with it a rebirth of the national arts.

From the Ming and Qing until just before Liberation, Chinese national folk dance went through a period where it was left to its own devices and had been devastated. But look, there is a drum regiment made up of artists following the army. On their waists hang small elliptical drums which they hit as they dance. What a stirring scene. Behind them comes a Yangge troupe formed of young men and women with coloured sashes tied to their waists. They advance twisting and swaying to the light dance steps of the Yangge as the sashes wave up and down in time to the lilting music. The boom of the drums and spirited dance steps merge with the excitement of the people celebrating Liberation to form a joyful atmosphere. No wonder this performance was named the "Victory Waist Drum".

Right back during the period of the Anti-Japanese War, in late 1942 and early 1943, artists and writers launched the "New Yangge Movement" at what was then the centre of the revolution, Yan'an. It advocated learning from folk song and dance arts, the "Drum Dance" and "Yangge Dance" being written after study of song and dance of Northern Shaanxi. Apart from performing these two joyful dances at large rallies, people also wrote Yangge dramas with singing and dancing which were based on this exuberant age-old folk dance. Examples are the "Brother and Sister Open Up Wasteland" reflecting the movement for increased production in the Liberated Areas and the "Husband and Wife Learn to Read" reflecting the anti-illiteracy campaign.

The "New Yangge Movement", which started in the Liberated Areas under the leadership of the Chinese Communist Party, also had an influence on those areas controlled by the Kuomintang then. At the time of the Anti-Japanese War the Kuomintang government moved its capital from Nanjing to Chongqing in Sichuan. The Chinese Communist Party Delegation led by Zhou Enlai and the Liaison Office of the Eighth Route Army were both stationed there. Thus the spirit of the "New Yangge Movement" was spread amongst progressive artists and writers in the Kuomintang areas via these organizations. "The Anti-Japanese Theatrical Propaganda Team" led and founded by Zhou Enlai himself was a group upholding progressive work in the performing arts in the Kuomintang areas. They made use of the "Dry Boat", "Small Cart" and other folk dance forms in song and dance arrangements which publicized resistance against the Japanese and the salvation of the country. The Yucai School set up by the famous educator Tao Xingzhi, took in many orphans who had lost their homes and been made destitute during the Anti-Japanese War and trained a considerable number of outstandingly talented people. The staff and teachers at the school went to the Liaison Office of the Eighth Route Army to study the "Yangge Dance" popular in Yan'an. They incorporated steps and dance poses from it to write and stage the "Ploughing and Sowing Dance", a depiction of peasant working life, and also turned another song popular in the Liberated Areas about a woman giving gifts to the Anti-Japanese Army, "Gift of Eggs from Old Mother Zhu", into a happy and lively dance performance. These dances circulated widely amongst progressive students in the Kuomintang areas.

In co-ordination with the Anti-Japanese and National Salvation Movement which was rapidly surging forwards, the famous Chinese dancer Wu Xiaobang adapted the songs of national salvation, "March of the Volunteers" and "Song of the Guerrillas", which enjoyed a countrywide vogue as dance performances. The "March of the Volunteers" with lyrics by the noted dramatist Tian Han and score by the famous musician Nie Er was originally a song from an outstanding thirties' film "Sons and Daughters of Storm". After Liberation it was adopted as the national anthem for the Pepole's Republic of China. Wu Xiaobang who was very young at the time used this extremely widely known piece in a dance arrangement. His passionate choreography, with its heroic military bearing, moved the hearts of countless patriots. The "Song of the Guerrillas" with lyrics and score by the famous musician He Luting was one of the most popular songs of the time. In the dance Wu Xiaobang gave a studied portrayal of the heroic figures of the guerrillas as they attacked the enemy with brave resourcefulness by melting in and out of thick woods. It was warmly praised. Wu Xiaobang saw with his own eyes how society actually was then under Kuomintang rule just as the great Tang poet Du Fu described in the line of a poem over 1,000 years earlier, "Behind the vermilion gates meat and wine go to waste while out on the road lie the bones of those frozen to death." These were the very conditions and sentiments which fired him to write the solo dance "Fire of Hunger": Under the window of a rich person's house with its scenes of debauchery, an impoverished man—a bag of bones on the verge of starvation—struggles for his life. With anguished cries he asks, what justice is there in life? Finally staring fixedly at the inequitable ways of the world, he dies nuring his hatred. The dances served to rouse the populace then and keep up morale.

Dai Ailian, a famous Chinese dancer who lived abroad for a long time returned home in 1940. The following year she went to the Yaoshan region in Guangxi to find out about and collect Yao dances. In 1945 she once again went to national minority districts in the area of Sichuan and Xikang (the name of an old province, now incorporated into the respective administrations of Sichuan and Tibet) taking students with her to collect national folk dances there. After returning to Chongqing, she produced and staged a show for border dances including the "Ba'an Xianzi", an arrangement based on the Tibetan folk "Xianzi Dance", and a female solo "Drums of the Yao" which utilized the Yao drum dances with certain improvements. Each had its own different national characteristics. "The Mute Gives a Piggyback to a Lunatic" was the fruit of Dai Ailian's studies of local traditional opera.

It is a Han folk dance performed by one person dressed up as two. The top half of the dancer is in female dresss. A pair of rolled up false legs are fitted as the lower limbs of a woman to the small of the back. The lower half of the body is in man's clothing with a false head and torso attached in front of the waist and chest as the upper part of a man. When danced, the actions must be co-ordinated so the movements of the dancer's legs fuse together with the trunk of the fake man and similarly the shaking of the upper half of the body must work as one with the fake woman's legs on the lower part of the back. The piece depicts a young couple. The wife, whose legs are paralyzed, is being carried outside on piggyback by her husband. On the way she picks a fresh flower from beside the road which she sticks in her hair by looking at her reflection in the water as they cross a bridge. In gazing at her own beautiful face, her attention wanders and she almost falls into the water. She quickly urges her husband to cross the bridge and they both hurry happily on their way. These details are, of course, all brought out in the dance movements. Dance shows in which one person plays two people date back several hundred years as a folk form in China. However, the dance qualities in Dai Ailian's performance of the "The Mute Gives a Piggyback to a Lunatic" are even stronger, with more beautiful imagery. These performances of dances from border areas attracted great interest and spread widely amongst young students.

In 1946 Wen Yiduo, the noted scholar and fighter for democracy in Kunming, the provincial capital of Yunnan, (he was assassinated on July 15th of the same year by a Kuomintang spy) along with progressive writers and artists organized their compatriots of Yi nationality from Guishan Mountains in Yunnan to go to Kunming and give a public performance of their national music and dance. In comment on this performance it was said that the "Axi, Moon Dance" "brimmed with such a great vitality and unquenchable enthusiasm that the whole audience must have been fired." Their show was also said to have "aroused people's confidence and strength in self-protection and portrayed their inviolate dignity".

Although it was before Liberation, progressive Chinese artists did some work in collecting and arranging national folk dance. However, such activities only gradually got going on a countrywide scale after the founding of the new China.

In 1949, the Literature and Art College at North China University, wrote and put on a large song and dance called "Long Live the People's Victory" in order to celebrate the opening of the Chinese People's Political Consultative Conference and to hail the setting up of the People's Republic of China. It incorporated a great deal of national folk music and dance—the creative fruit of many years of learning from folk arts by musicians and artists throughout the country. Included were the stirring "Drum Dance", lively "Large Yangge", beautifully evocative "Lotus Lamp", exuberant "Xinjiang Dance" and the "Tibetan Dance" which was a riot of colour. Artists utilized artistic forms created by the peoples of various nationalities in composing this song of praise which gave expression to the great vitality of the people's aspirations. It was most impressive.

In the early fifties, the Central Visiting Group organized by the Party and government went to national minority areas in border areas to convey their greetings to people there who had been badly suppressed in the old society. Musicians and dancers accompanying them eagerly learned traditional songs and dances wherever they went from their compatriots in national minorities. On National Day in 1951 the large format song and dance "Great Unity of the Peoples" had its première at

Beijing. It showed scenes of people from national minorities enjoying themselves singing and dancing to their hearts' content on the Tian An Men Square. People saw various styles of dance such as Han, Uygur, Mongolian, Tibetan, Yao, Miao and that of the Gaoshan people from Taiwan in this piece. It was a review of the achievements of professional musicians and dancers in learning from the national folk art tradition.

The Central National Song and Dance Troupe established in 1952, took the "Great Unity of the Peoples" on tour all over China to great effect. The same troupe together with the Arts Department at the Central Institute for Nationalities did a lot of work in collecting, arranging and creating national folk dances as well as in the training of people talented in music and dance from all nationalities.

From 1953-1957, the Ministry of Culture held several festivals: the First National Folk Music and Dance Festival; the National Mass Amateur Theatrical Festival; National Professional Groups' Music and Dance Festival; the Second National Folk Music and Dance Festival. Many excellent national folk music and dance pieces as well as outstanding performing talent emerged at these national festivals.

In the space of a few years, a large number of folk dances on the verge of extinction or already extinct were unearthed and revised to gain a new lease of life thanks to the efforts of numerous dancers. Pieces such as the "Dragon Dance", "Lion Dance", "Carp Dance", "Dry Boat", "Yangge" and "Flower Drum" were originally dances for the masses own entertainment created by the Han in the course of recreational activities at traditional festivals. They are several hundred or even thousand years old. However, before Liberation, such folk dances were not "deemed elegant" and did not receive the attention they deserved. Some degenerated into a source of livelihood for itinerant peasants. Now not only have they been staged in the capital but rearranged and improved on by the dancers and performed abroad where they were praised by audiences.

Since the establishment of the new China, national organizations, local bodies in provinces, cities and autonomous areas as well as the Chinese People's Liberation Army have set up song and dance troupes one after another. The ranks of dancers have quickly expanded and the artistic level continued to improve so the work of carrying on and spreading the national folk dance tradition has developed in depth and breadth. A large number of dance pieces in a folk style typically Chinese have emerged and proved highly popular.

Han folk dance has broken new ground. Take for example the "Lotus Dance" derived from the Northern Shaanxi folk dance "Lotus Lantern" which pays tribute to peace and happiness: A group of young girls, their shoulders draped in fine gauze, wear lotus leaf hoops beneath their long dresses. Four brightly coloured lotuses stretch upwards from the edges. With smooth, lithe footwork consisting of broken steps the dancers evoke the way lotuses drift and move on the surface of the water. Its unconventional beauty makes it entertaining as well as pleasing to the eye. "Flying Celestials", a work which took its inspiration from the well-known figures of flying celestials and celestial entertainers on murals at Dunhuang in Gansu is distinctive in style. The performers wear ancient costumes. Silk sashes about seven metres long swirl between their arms. Its many postures give it a refined yet flowing feel as if a wind-borne goddess is sowing seeds of happiness to the people of the world. The first dance to draw on material from murals at Dunhuang, it is an enchanting piece with a well-knit structure and smooth actions. The "Lotus Dance" and "Flying Celestials" are both artistic gems created in the fifties by the noted dancer

Dai Ailian.

"Picking Tea and Catching Butterflies" a creative arrangement based on the "Tea-Picking Lantern" from Fujian, depicts a group of girls who go into the mountains to pick tea. On the way back from their work they find a large, beautiful butterfly (the butterfly is tied to the tip of a springy rattan cane held by a boy). They gather round and play at trying to catch it. It is a fresh and lively piece with a zest for life. "Racing Donkey" is an other arrangement which makes use of material from Northern Shaanxi folk dance. A young peasant couple carrying their child home to the woman's parents is portrayed. The female character has a donkey's head and body attached in front of her at the waist and behind the hindlegs and tail. Her legs are covered round with cloth so it looks as if she is riding on donkey back with the child in her arms. The "donkey" trots along or slowly ambles or sometimes gets stuck in the mud. The husband follows in support at one side and ends up pulling the donkey out of the mud as they go happily on their way. The dance is full of human interest from the Northern Shaanxi countryside. The "Red Silk Dance", an arrangement in which forms from the traditional "Sash Dance" are used, owes its success to its fire and energy: A group of young men and women carrying torches come on stage dancing "Yangge" steps. With a wave of their hands the torches turn into long red silks which twist and swirl in the air in figures of eight, spiral shapes or waves. Suddenly the actors leap up high and with a flick form the red silks into a large circle. The actresses then jump inside it.... The whole stage seems to flicker with flames of joy.

The "Song of a Good Harvest" which draws on folk dance material from the south of the Yangtze area, brims with the joy of the peasants after a bumper harvest. The bluff, forthright dance movements give it a simple, wholesome artistic style rich in local flavour. The folk dance "Flower Drum Lantern" popular on the banks of the River Huaihe in Anhui has a more complete structure now that it has been arranged and worked on by dancers. The group dance "Large Scene" opens to the noisy sound of gongs and drums. The elated dance movements with their military vigour merge bits from martial arts and acrobatics inspiring all who see it. The mixed pas de deux "Small Scene" has charm and wit, often raising gales of laughter from the audience. Both "Flying to Take Luding Bridge", a portrayal of the battle life of the Red Army on the Long March, and the "Immortal Warrior" depicting the heroic deeds of Huang Jiguang, a martyr in the Chinese People's Volunteers, are arrangements based on life in the army which make use of classical dance and mat skills (mainly referring to all kinds of rolling actions). They have both been very successful.

National minority folk dances are even more rich and varied. The "Peacock Dance" is an age-old traditional dance of the Dai people. It was originally danced by a man wearing a costume and headdress in the form of a peacock. The women's group dance of the same name is an arrangement based on it. The performers wear light dancing costumes with distinctive national features. The hems of the skirts bear a beautiful pattern of peacock feathers. By means of graceful dancing poses, various movements of the peacock are portrayed such as fanning its feathers, shaking its wings, walking and drinking. A lyrical piece. Tibetan folk dances such as the 'Tap Dance", "Xianzi Dance" and "Bell and Drum Dance" were made use of in writing the "Reba on the Grasslands". Included are evocative passages of great beauty when the long sleeves are slowly twirled as well as wild and unrestrained group dancing in which the men shake bronze bells and the women strike flat drums. Solo performances of special skills are interleaved as well so it is very lively. Creative arrangements of material from Yi national folk dances such as "The Happy Luosuo" and the "Axi Moon Dance" portray the jubilant feelings of the Yi people after Liberation. The "Straw Hat Dance" distilled from the life of the Li people is rich in their national dance style, a lively and carefree work of moving beauty. There are also the Mongolian dances "Tending Horses" and "Wild Goose Dance" performed by the famous dancer Jia Zuoguang; the "Long Drum Dance" performed by the well-known Korean dancer Cui Meishan; the "Cup and Bowl Dance" performed by the Mongolian dancer Modegema; "Picking Grapes" performed by the Uygur dancer Ayitula; and the "Gauze Sash Dance" performed by the Tatar dancer Zuohala.

All of these Han and national minority artistic works based on tradition and containing innovations have been active on stage in China as well as having been performed abroad many times. A number of pieces have taken prizes at international competitions so winning honour for the people and country of China.

Folk dance disciplines have been set up in dance schools throughout the land. Many experienced dance teachers have been very successful in collecting, revising and arranging national folk dance material. Fairly thorough studies have been carried out on those classical dances preserved in Chinese traditional opera in particular so as to help restore and develop the traditional dance system of the Chinese people. Many old time performing artists in the world of traditional opera have made a great contribution in this respect.

In the mid-fifties, Chinese dancers created a national dance with a distinctive style based on their study of national tradition and the use of foreign dance forms as reference. It was pioneering work in the history of Chinese dance. The *Precious Lotus Lamp* is the first large-scale Chinese dance drama. Its theme is a story from legend which enjoys wide circulation amongst the Han people. As long as 600 or 700 years ago it had already been put on as a traditional opera, and in recent times this traditional piece has figured in both Beijing and local operas. The story relates how the goddess Sanshengmu fell in love with a young scholar from the mortal world, Liu Yanchang. Her way was barred by a General of Heaven, the god Erlang, but by relying on the Precious Lotus Lamp she beat him, came down to the mortal world and was married to Liu Yanchang. Over a year later, just as friends and relatives were celebrating the hundredth day since the birth of their son Chenxiang, the god Erlang ordered the barking Hound of Heaven to steal the Precious Lotus Lamp first and he then burst into the Liu house, carried off Sanshengmu and imprisoned her beneath Mount Huashan. In the confusion the great God of Thunder, ready to fight in a just cause, saved their son, brought him up to adulthood and taught him martial art skills. A dozen or so years later, Chenxiang, now in his early youth, made straight for Mount Huashan and had a great battle with the generals of Heaven guarding it under the god Erlang. He wrested back the Precious Lotus Lamp, split open Huashan and released his mother. Finally Liu Yanchang rushed up and husband and wife and father and son were reunited. Zhao Qing who played Sanshengmu is a quite outstanding dancer trained in the new China. She gives an exquisite portrayal of Sanshengmu's character, gentle and full of tenderness yet resolute and decisive. At the same time she also has quite a full grasp of the rules of expression and skills in Chinese classical dance. Folk dances from many areas such as the "Flower Drum Lantern", "Big Head Dance" and

"Dragon Dance" are also incorporated in the dance drama. These dance scenes are all arranged according to the requirements of plot development and merge as one with the tenor of the classical dancing in the piece creating a novel effect.

Some quite outstanding national dance dramas emerged in the wake of the *Precious Lotus Lamp*. Examples are a dance drama called the *Dagger Society* which has as its theme the struggle of a rebel unit in Shanghai against the Qing government and imperialists during the Taiping Revolution; the dance drama *Five Red Clouds* with the revolutionary struggle of the Yi people from the Wuzhi Mountains on Hainan Island off Guangdong as its subject matter; or another dance drama the *Manluo Flower* which has Miao folk legends portraying unwavering love as its subject. The advent of this first group of dances laid the foundation for the development of a Chinese national dance drama.

In 1964 to celebrate the 15th anniversary of the founding of New China, Premier Zhou Enlai himself was in charge of organizing more than 3,000 professional and amateur artists in the writing and staging of a large-format music and dance epic called the *East Is Red*. It briefly depicted important stages of the Chinese revolution: the old disaster-ridden China; the birth of the Chinese Communist Party; the Northern Expedition; Land Revolution; the Long March by the Red Army; the Zunyi Conference; the Anti-Japanese War; the War of Liberation; the founding of New China. Besides incorporating works of music and dance representative of each historical period, it went even further by bringing together many outstanding national songs and dances written since Liberation in an imposing and deeply moving epic with strong appeal.

Just as Chinese dance operations were flourishing, disaster fell. The so called "cultural revolution" which started in 1966, created a catastrophe unprecedented in history. For the 10 years it lasted, literary and artistic circles suffered the worst. The "gang of four" with Jiang Qing as ringleader completely negated achievements in the work in literary and artistic fields during the 17 years from the founding of the People's Republic of China. Large numbers of leading cadres in literary and artistic circles, famous performers and folk artistes were blamed for all sorts of crimes and dealt a cruel blow, many being persecuted to death. National folk music and dance were vilified as "unhealthy", "pornographic" and "decadent music". Traditional festivals of the various nationalities along with their festive dance activities were all regarded as being "feudal and backward" and thus abolished. Many gifted choreographer-directors and performers were sent down to the countryside for long periods to take part in simple manual labour. They had no chance to perform their art and were even deprived of the right to practise their skills. For 10 whole years, the development of Chinese national folk dance stagnated.

In October 1976, the "gang of four" and the feudal, fascist dictatorship they implemented were smashed, the Chinese people and their arts being liberated for the second time. Dancers who had been deprived of 10 years of their artistic life now took up the work of reviving and developing national folk dance with redoubled vigour to make good the losses brought about by the past catastrophe. In the space of just a few years, dance troupes all over the country once again staged excellent programmes written since the founding of the People's Republic of China and also wrote and performed many new works which had a distinctive national style. Some were of an even higher standard than previously.

To celebrate the 30th anniversary of the founding of the People's Republic of China in 1979, the Ministry of Culture held a large-scale theatrical festival. It was a nationwide review of all types of theatrical pieces in which there appeared highly creative dances and dance dramas. The folk dance drama *Rain of Flowers on the Silk Road* produced and staged by the Gansu Song and Dance Troupe was particularly outstanding. By the use of novel yet age-old dancing poses and various dance styles a song of praise to the friendship between the people of China and abroad was woven. The story takes place more than 1,000 years ago during the Tang Dynasty. An artisan called Zhang the Miraculous Painter saved Yinusi, a Parsian merchant, who had collapsed amid the sand and wind on the ancient Silk Road linking the north west of China with the Middle East. However Zhang's only daughter Yingniang, was carried off by bandits. Several years later Zhang saw her, reduced to a common song and dance girl, in the market at Dunhuang athrong with foreign merchants. Yinusi bought back her freedom with jewellery thus reuniting father and daughter. A corrupt official Shi Cao wanted to seize Yingniang for himself so Zhang sent her off with Yinusi to far away Persia. Shi Cao punished Zhang by making him paint murals at the Mogao Caves in chains. The Military Governor for the Shaanxi and Gansu area went there to pay his devotions. He so admired Zhang's drawings that he gave him back his freedom. Soon afterwards, Yinusi acting as an emissary from Persia to the Tang court was returning with Yingniang to Dunhuang when they were stopped on the way by bandits. After this was discovered by Zhang he lit a beacon fire to raise the alarm. Yinusi and Yingniang were saved but Zhang was shot dead on the beacon tower by the bandits. At a friendly meeting of 27 countries at Dunhuang, Yingniang put on makeup and gave a presentation performance which she used to reveal to the Military Governor how Shi Cao had colluded with the bandits in their wrong-doings. The Military Governor ordered the evil-doers to be punished and from then on the Silk Road, symbol of the friendship between the peoples of China and abroad, was trouble free.

After much deliberation, the director and actors in *Rain of Flowers on the Silk Road* researched murals and sculptures in over 400 caves covering a period of more than 1,000 years from the Southern and Northern Dynasties up to the Yuan at the Mogao Caves in Dunhuang and the Yulin Caves in Anxi. They made a meticulous study of the large range of dancing poses in the ancient murals and thus came to understand the styles and rules of expression which emerged. By investigating what the movements must have been like before they took the form of static poses and the changes that could have taken place after they had taken form, they established structural links between them in light of the rules of movement in classical dance. Thus these motionless dance postures were resurrected in a dance idiom and combinations which had both life and feeling. They went on to create the distinctive "Dunhuang style" of dance. The familiar figure of "Flying Celestials" from murals at Dunhuang, was transformed into the beautiful "Flying Celestial Dance" of the prelude. Several actresses soar across a sky swirling with mist in an enchanting dance. Yingniang's solo "Playing the *Pipa* Backwards" absorbed dance forms from celestial entertainers playing the *pipa* backward in the "Scripture Story Painting" series at the Mogao Caves. While painting the caves Zhang dreams of the Heavenly Palace and sees his daughter Yingniang dancing with a group of goddesses in a reproduction of music and dance scenes from murals at Dunhuang. *Rain of Flowers on the Silk Road* was praised by the dance world and audiences alike.

The dance drama *Zhaoshutun and Nan-*

muruona performed by the Dai Autonomous Prefecture Song and Dance Ensemble of Xishuangbanna, Yunnan, is an arrangement based on the narrative poem "Zhaoshutun" which has circulated amongst the Dai for many years. Long, long ago King Mengbanjia held a ceremony to select a wife for his son Zhaoshutun. Many young Dai girls came forward as candidates. An important minister called Xina wanted to marry his own daughter to the prince but met with the prince's refusal. The prince went hunting alone by the Golden Lake and fell in love with the Peacock Princess Nanmuruona who had flown there to bathe. Just as the marriage ceremony was being held, a neighbouring country invaded so the prince set out on an expedition to ward them off. Xina made use of this to falsely accuse Nanmuruona of bringing misfortune to the nation and had her driven away. Zhaoshutun returned in triumph to find her gone and exposed Xina and the sorcerer's plot. Setting off in search of his sweetheart, after all kinds of hardship and dangers, he finally brought Nanmuruona back from the Kingdom of the Peacocks. They became man and wife. The Dai are one of the national minorities in China with an outstanding tradition of dance. The entire dance drama is in a pure and fresh style with rich national colouring like a beautiful lyric poem.

The fact that the Tang Princess Wencheng went to far of Tibet to marry Songzanganbu thus furthering unity and friendship between the Han and Tibetan has been used many times in the 1,000 years since as the theme for works of literature and art. The dance drama *Princess Wencheng* is another arrangement based on this event. Chen Ailian who plays Princess Wencheng is a quite talented dancer who won the gold medal for her performance of the classical Chinese dance *A Moonlit Spring Night by the River of Flowers* at the Eighth World Youth Festival 18 years ago. She has also played the female lead in dance dramas such as *Zhang Yu and Qionglian* and the *Fish Beauty*. She has excellent innate dance qualities and a good grounding in basics with a fairly comprehensive technique. She excels at expressing the characters' feelings through her postures and movements. Having been through the 10 catastrophic years she is once again performing so people can see she has lost nothing of her charm. Zhang Minxin, one of the choreographers and directors of *Princess Wencheng* is a highly talented female choreographer and director who is both strict and thorough. Her maiden work *Hua'er and the Young Man* was a national hit. When she took part in directing the dance drama *Fish Beauty*, she came up with such brilliant pieces as "The Snake Dance" or "The Coral Dance" which remain standards for dance troupes even today.

Dance pieces derived from national folk dance formed the greater part of the performance in tribute to the 30th anniversary of national Day. They were just too beautiful for words. For example there was "As an Everlasting Memento" written with material from Tibetan dance which was an expression of people's deep longing for the late Premier Zhou Enlai; or the comic children's dance "Looking at the Lamp" created from forms in the Han folk "Changing the Straw Hat" from Sichuan. By depicting the disgusting behaviour of the "gang of four" through exaggeration, it voiced the people's loathing for them; the "Water Keepers", a work of moving beauty, was written on the basis of Korean national dance. The group of lovely young girls in green costumes were the personification of grain seedlings growing to sturdy maturity thanks to assiduous watering by the "Water Keepers"; "A Memorable Water Sprinkling Festival" reflects a traditional Dai festival described in that nationality's own dance idiom. It depicts the moving scene of Premier Zhou Enlai spending the Water Sprinkling Festival when still alive with Dai people at Xishuangbanna in Yunnan.

In May 1980, a Staff and Workers Amateur Theatrical Festival with sections for provinces, cities and autonomous regions was held in Beijing. In June the same year another one for peasant amateur arts took place. These two festivals enabled audiences in the capital to see dance arts which had sprung directly from the people. Items performed by peasants made an especially deep impression with their local flavour. The "Hundred Leaf Dragon" put on by peasants from Zhejiang is an age-old traditional dance. As the curtain rose, lotuses could be seen floating amongst lotus leaves. In a trice, the lotus flowers jerked apart to link up into a scaly hundred leaf dragon which snaked and twisted in exact co-ordination with the movements of the dragon dancer. It was as if it was a real life dragon flying through the clouds. The "Drum Yangge" performed by peasants from Shandong had a spirited gusto. Some danced beating drums and others twirling parasols. The dance actions flowed into each other yet remained flexible too. This dance which has circulated for many years amongst Han in Shandong was well received.

In August, 1980, the Ministry of Culture and the Association of Chinese Dancers held a competition for solo, duo and trio dances at Dalian in Liaoning. Some outstanding works of national dance which caught people's attention appeared. "The Battle Drum of Golden Mountain" was a trio dance depicting the famous heroine of the Northern Song, Liang Hongyu, beating a drum in the fight against Tartar troops. The choreographers made a thorough study of the dancing, armed fighting movements and methods of presentation of "women's military roles" in traditional Chinese opera. They carefully designed a plot and dance combinations which developed around the battle drum. With a valiant air, Liang Hongyu and her sons—two young generals—played the battle drum to direct the fighting. She jumped up onto the drum to make a reconnaisance and was suddenly hit in the arm by an arrow. Putting up with the pain she ordered her son to pull it out to once again beat the drum with flailing arms, urging on the officers and men to kill the enemy bravely and secure victory. Extremely difficult yet beautiful dance movements were used to express these details. Liang Hongyu performed a "forward flip" onto the drum surface which was only just over a metre in diameter. After being wounded she again executed a "back flip" and jumped down. In the final fierce battle, Liang Hongyu and her sons surrounded the drum on three sides to perform a series of "rapid turns" (a rapid spin with the body at an angle) as they beat the drum. Such demanding performances were really thrilling and gave a powerful depiction of the desperate battle between the heroes and the enemy. The main dance director, Pang Zhiyang, has a great deal of creative experience. For a long time now he has devoted himself to study and research into the tradition of national and folk dancing arts. He has written many outstanding dance works.

"Catching Fish" was a duo derived from the Dai folk "Fish Dance". A pretty "little fish" was swimming carefree in the water. An old fisherman groped for it with his hands in the water as the "little fish" darted here and there trying to hide. It was caught. The lovely "little fish" had to resign itself to being led home.... Suddenly, it wriggled out of the old fisherman's hands and slipped back into the water again. The piece has a happy, relaxed appeal full of vitality and Dai national folk dance style. Another Dai female solo dance "Water" was performed by the noted dancer of Dai nationality, Dao Meilan. It portrayed a scene common in life: a young Dai girl arrives at the banks of a river carrying two buckets across the shoulder. She stares at the fresh, cool running water and letting down her head of thick black hair rinses it. She then jumps in to let the flowing water wash away her work fatigue. Having climbed back up on the bank she shakes her beautiful, long hair. Spinning round she puts it up in the bun characteristic of young Dai girls. The entire dance is in a simple, unadorned arrangement which in combination with Dao Meilan's exquisite performance leaves a quiet, graceful impression.

The three-person "Monkey Drum" written with material from the Miao folk dance of the same name and incorporating skills and techniques from "Changing Faces" in Sichuan Opera, is an entertaining piece. "Seeing Brother Off to Battle", a duo, makes use of dance steps from the Northern Shaanxi folk Yangge with additional improvements and changes. There are also other examples such as the Korean "Golden Festival Cymbals" and the Uygur "My Rewafu", all outstanding dances with distinctive national features which made an appearance in the competition.

The National Minority Theatrical Festival held in Beijing by the Ministry of Culture and the State Nationalities Affairs Commission in September and October 1980 was of especial significance. It goes without saying that delegates from national minorities had participated in all previous theatrical festivals since the founding of the People's Republic of China. However, this was the first time in 30 years that a national festival had been organized solely for national minority art. Delegates from all the 55 minority nationalities took part in the performance putting on twenty-one music, dance, opera and drama pieces in all. It was the stage début for some of them. All the items were characterized by a distinctive national style and included developments and innovations based on tradition. The Tibetan dance "Happy Linka" was a creative arrangement of Tibetan folk "Tap Dance" forms.

"Linka" means "park". A group of young Tibetans are depicted dancing happily in a park to the sound of lingering music. All of a sudden the music stops and only the regular powerful sound of tap dancing, varying in strength and speed, can be heard on stage. The young people's cheerful frame of mind is brought out in a highly rhythmic way.

"A Piggyback for the Bride" is a narrative dance based on the dances and customs of Yi nationality. On the day when a young Yi couple are married, the bride arranges for several unmarried girl friends to wait at her house. The groom also asks some of his bachelor friends to come and meet the bride. By an old custom, visiting the bride is not such a simple matter. Her friends crowd together and splash the visitors with water, beat them, smear makeup on their faces and prevent them getting near the bride. The young visitors just have to dodge out of the way not being allowed to retaliate. After some lively fun and games, they overcome all the difficulties and help the bridegroom to eventually carry the bride off home on his back. The choreographer Huang Shi lived amongst the Yi for a long time and was fully conversant with their music, dance and customs which he cleverly combined to create this piece. With distinctive national features, the dance idiom is lively and carefree. The entire performance brims with a joyful exuberance from beginning to end.

Guangxi dance workers studied a wealth of historical data based on the Huashan Cliff Murals in writing the "Battle Drum of Huashan". It is a personification of the spirit with which the forefathers of the Zhuang bravely united together to fight. The dance idiom draws on the Zhuang traditional "Shigong Dance", "Carrying-Pole Dance" and "Bronze Drum Dance" with some additional improvements and changes. Its style of raw primitive beauty can be said to bring the ancient Huashan Cliff Murals back to life in some ways.

The "Goat-Picking Dance" of the Kazaks from Xinjiang presents a sports entertainment from a Kazak folk festival in an extremely lively dance form. A crowd of young men vie to catch a goat as they charge along on horseback. The dancers posture and movements are wild and fervent with different dance idioms being used to portray various kinds of prancing and galloping.

There are other national minority dances which have only been unearthed recently by dance workers such as the Yi "Bronze Drum Dance". Originally it was an ancient traditional dance custom prevalent in the area of Yunnan. Whenever the Dagong Festival was held (around the end of July every year) — a traditional Yi festival to celebrate good harvests and pray for fine weather — or there was a marriage, building of a new house or death of an old person, all the men and women of the village, young and old, had to gather together to beat bronze drums and dance the "Qili" (i.e., a celebration dance). The custom dates back several hundred years. However during the 10 years of catastrophe, customs and cultural traditions of the national minorities were all regarded as "backward" and "corrupting public morals" so were discontinued under the ban. The bronze drums beloved by the Yi people were buried deep underground, the people no longer being allowed to dance the "Qili". To participate in the countrywide National Minority Theatrical Festival, dancers from Yunnan went right down amongst the Yi for a quiet chat and dispelled their misgivings. They dug up the bronze drums and danced the "Qili" all night long in the bright moonlight. On the basis of this visit the dancers wrote the "Bronze Drum Dance", a dance with a lively rhythm which places the emphasis on twisting and swaying movements. To the beat of the drums, the Yi people's happiness is brought out in the robustly beautiful dance steps.

The original manuscript of "Tending the Lion" from the Tibetan nationality area of Gansu Province was only unearthed recently, preserved in a temple. A pair of dancers in goat skins play a snowy-white lion. It crouches down with body raised, sometimes shaking its head and mane, cocking its head and tail or lies on the ground licking its coat, docile and lovable. This age-old dance died out long ago. More than 1,000 years earlier the great Tang poet Bai Juyi gave a lively description of a lion dance from Xiliang (modern Wuwei in Gansu) in his poem "Xiliang Arts". Possibly "Tending the Lion" is in the same tradition as the lion dance which circulated in the Gansu area long, long ago.

The dances of the Deng people who inhabit border areas of Tibet are in an uninhibited and vigorous style. The dance for two "The Deng People and the Morning Glory" portrays their hunting life and pure love. "Springtime for the Xiaerba" a group dance reflecting the life of the Xiaerba people who live on the frontier of China and Nepal contains gentle dance poses with the characteristics of Eastern dance. A refreshing experience. "A Flower Blooms on a Goat's Horn", a dance of the Qiang nationality, features twisting and shaking of the body as well as swinging of the ornamental shoulder tassels. This female solo dance has something unique about it. The tradition of Manchu folk dance was lost long ago. The "Mangshi Kongqi" performed at the festival is an ancient folk dance arrangement drawn from scattered historical records about the characteristics of Manchu dance movements.

During the early years of the People's Republic of China, the Chinese Communist Party and Central People's Government worked out a policy for the development of national minority art and literature which enjoyed certain success. However during the 10 years of catastrophe, the nationality policy was totally destroyed by Lin Biao, Jiang Qing and their cohorts. National minority art and literature was particularly badly hit. Today, people have seen large numbers of dazzling shows staged at national theatrical festivals throughout the country. Even limiting the discussion to the spectacular dances touched on in the text, it is more than enough to fill us with enthusiasm. This proves that popular art has great vitality and cannot be destroyed by any force at all. This festival marked the revival of Chinese national minority art and literature as well as their entry into a completely new stage of development.

For the past 30 years the continuation and development of Chinese national folk art have followed a tortuous route. Judging by what has been achieved in the last four years, I am quite confident that so long as we persevere with the artistic policy of "letting a hundred flowers blossom" we can overcome all obstacles on our path forward and achieve greater and greater success.

中国舞蹈史话

王克芬 著

*

外文出版社出版
（中国北京百万庄路24号）
外文印刷厂印刷
中国国际图书贸易总公司
（中国国际书店）发行
北京399信箱
1985年（16开）第一版
编号：（英）7050—56
00520
7—E—1809P

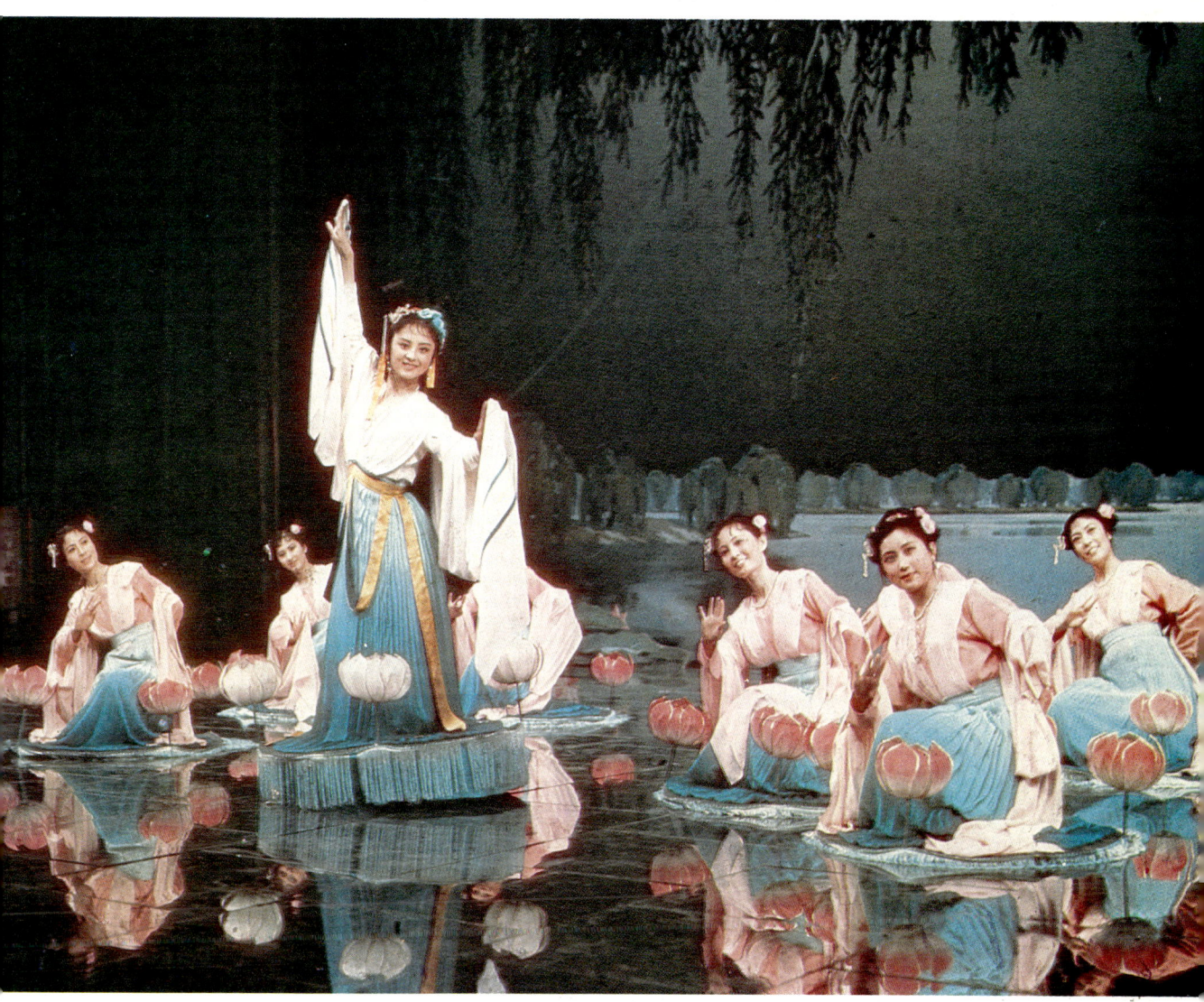

1. The "Lotus Dance" (Han).

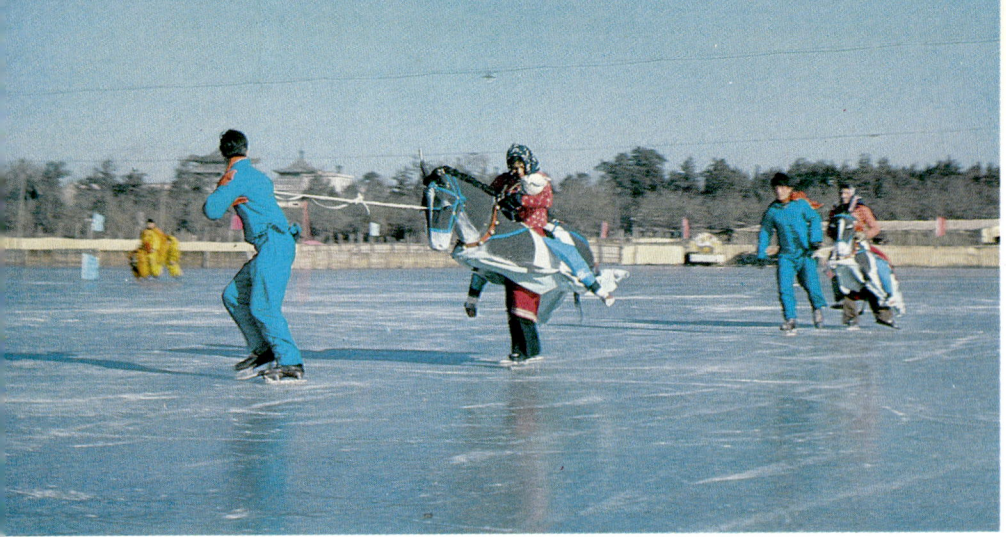

2. "Racing Donkeys" performed on ice (Han).

3. "Red Silk Dance" (Han).

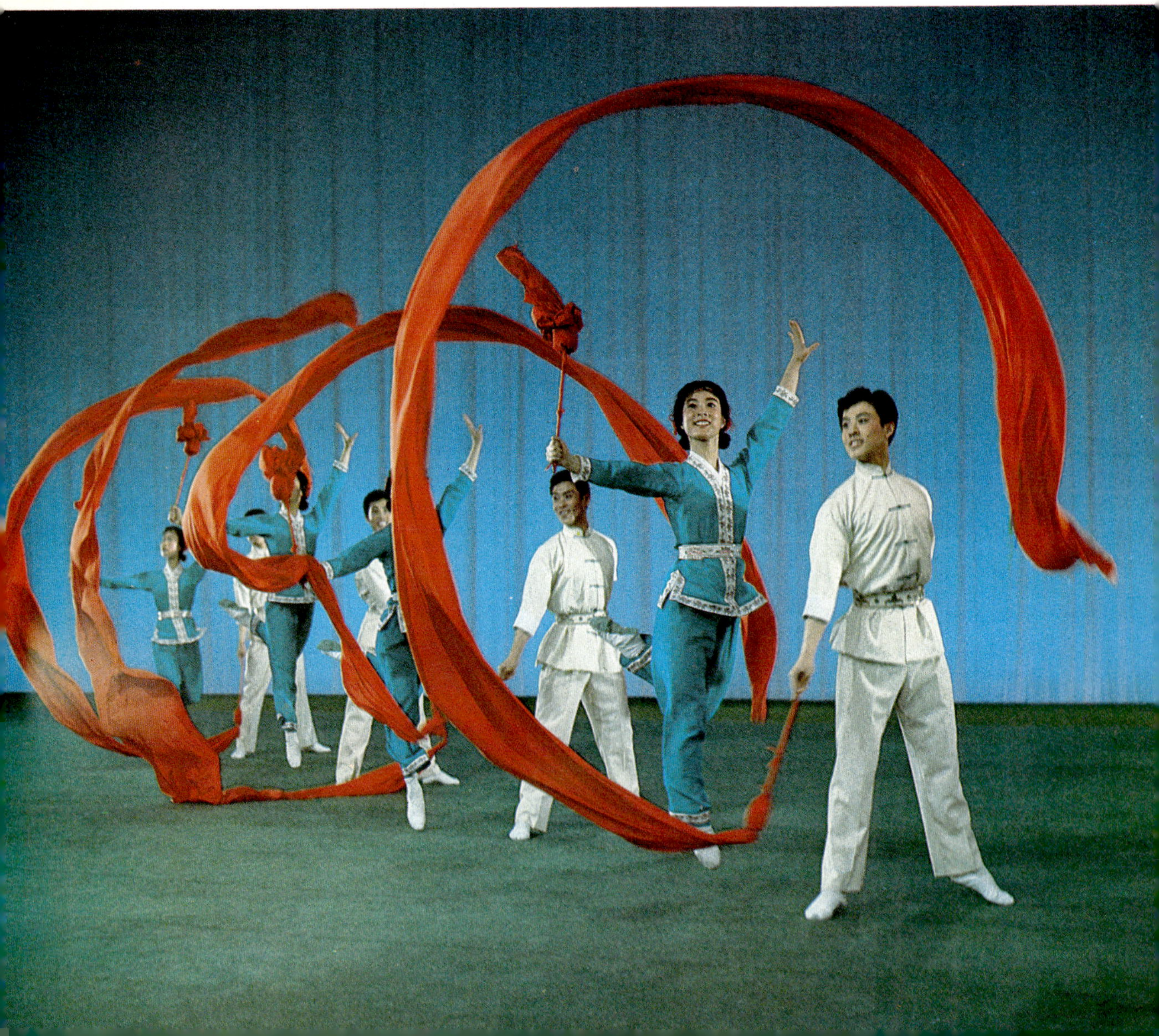

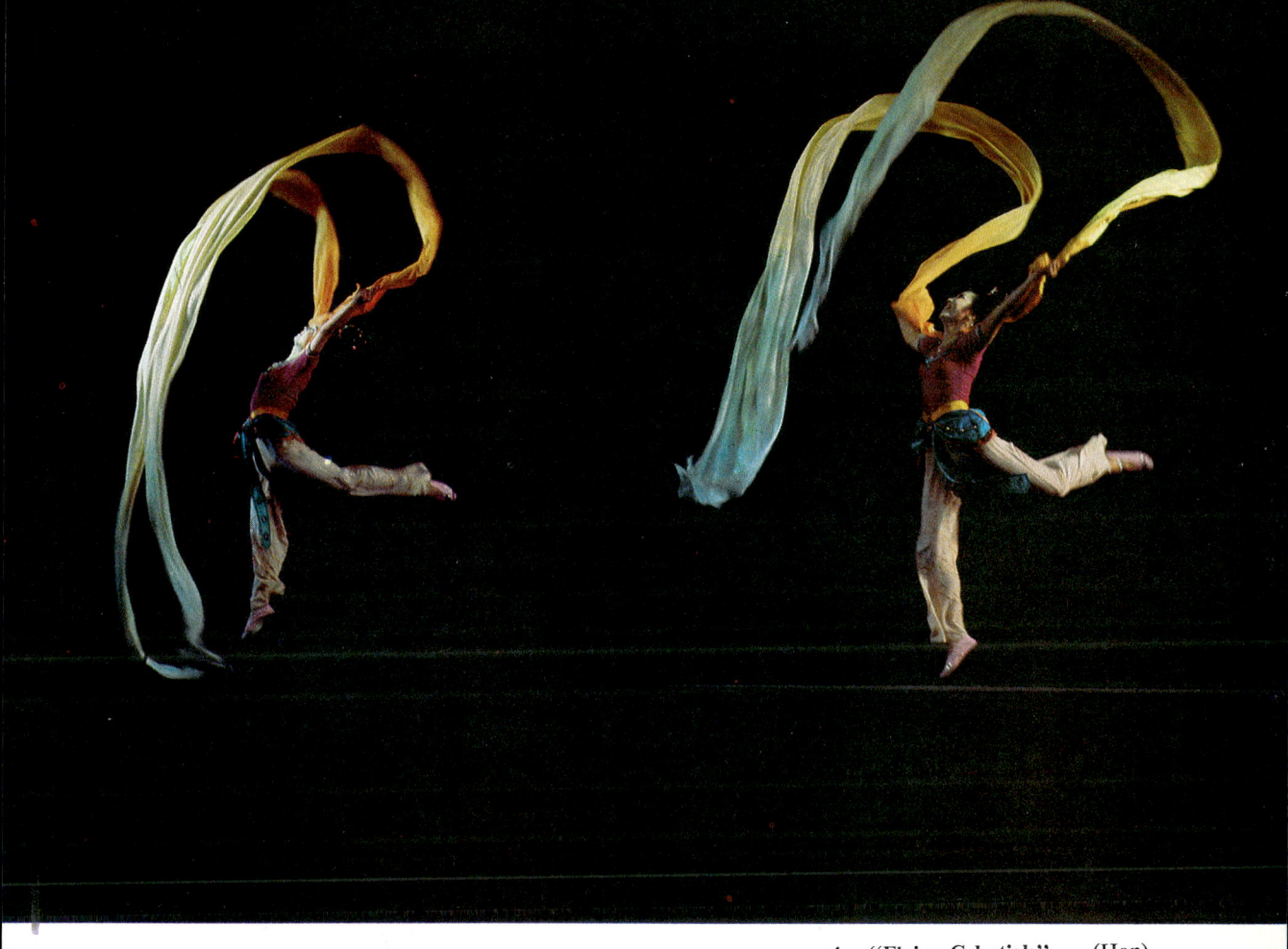

4. "Flying Celestials" (Han).

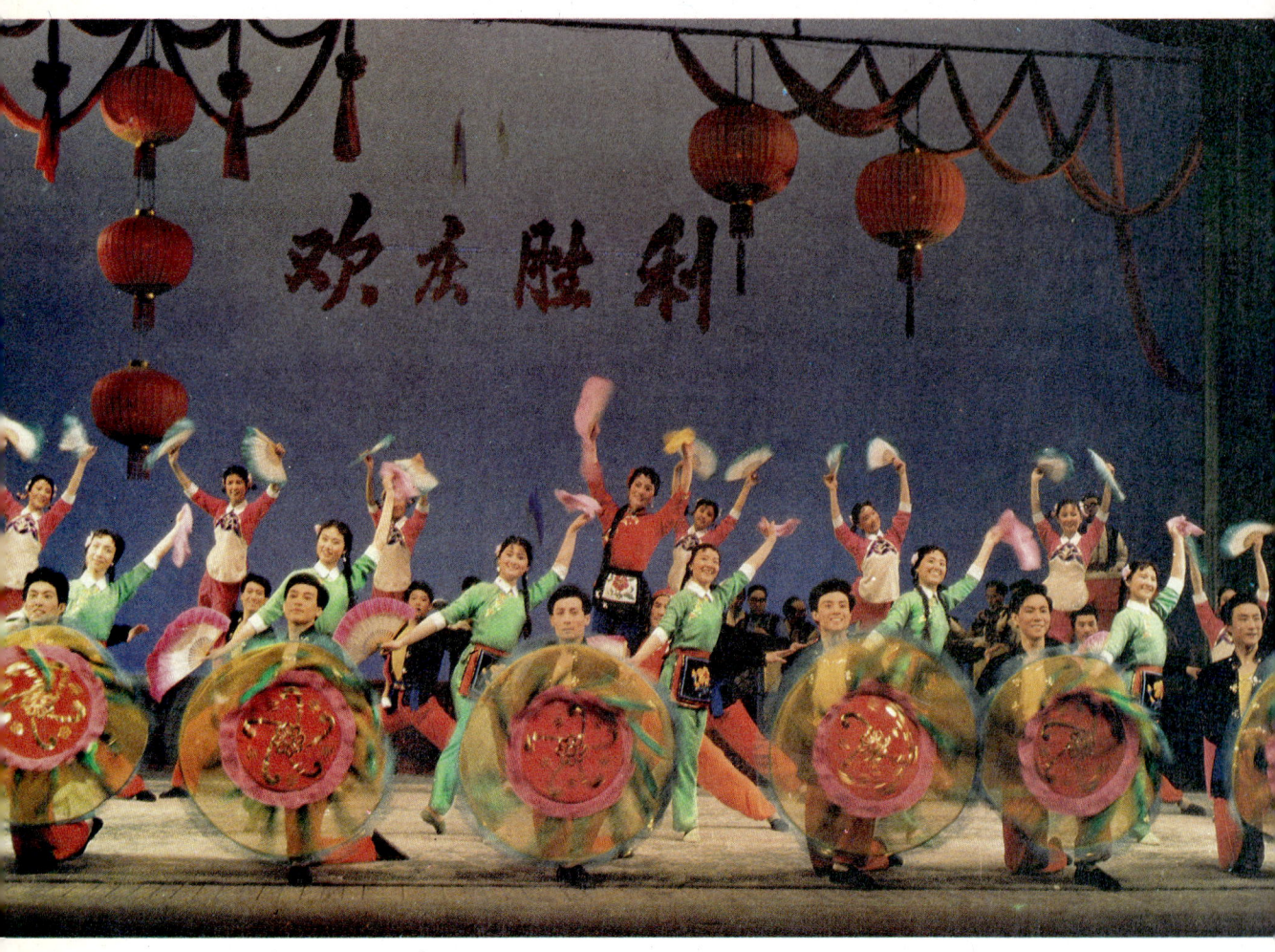

5. "Flower Drum Lantern"   (Han).

6. "Peacock Dance" (Dai).

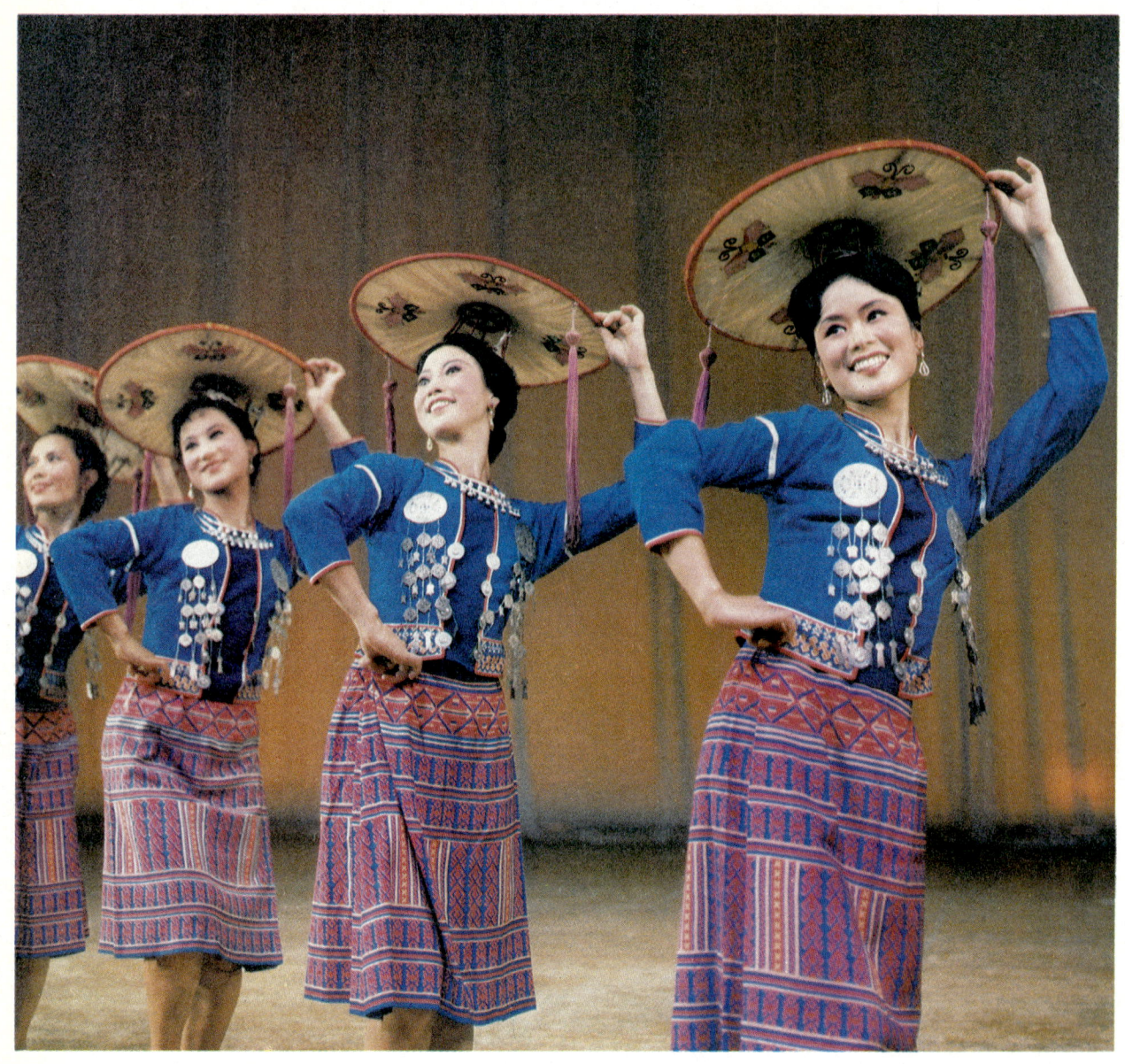

7. "Straw Hat Dance"   (Li).

8. The Korean dancer Cui Meishan performing the "Long Drum Dance".

9. The Mongolian dancer Modegema performing the "Cup and Bowl Dance".

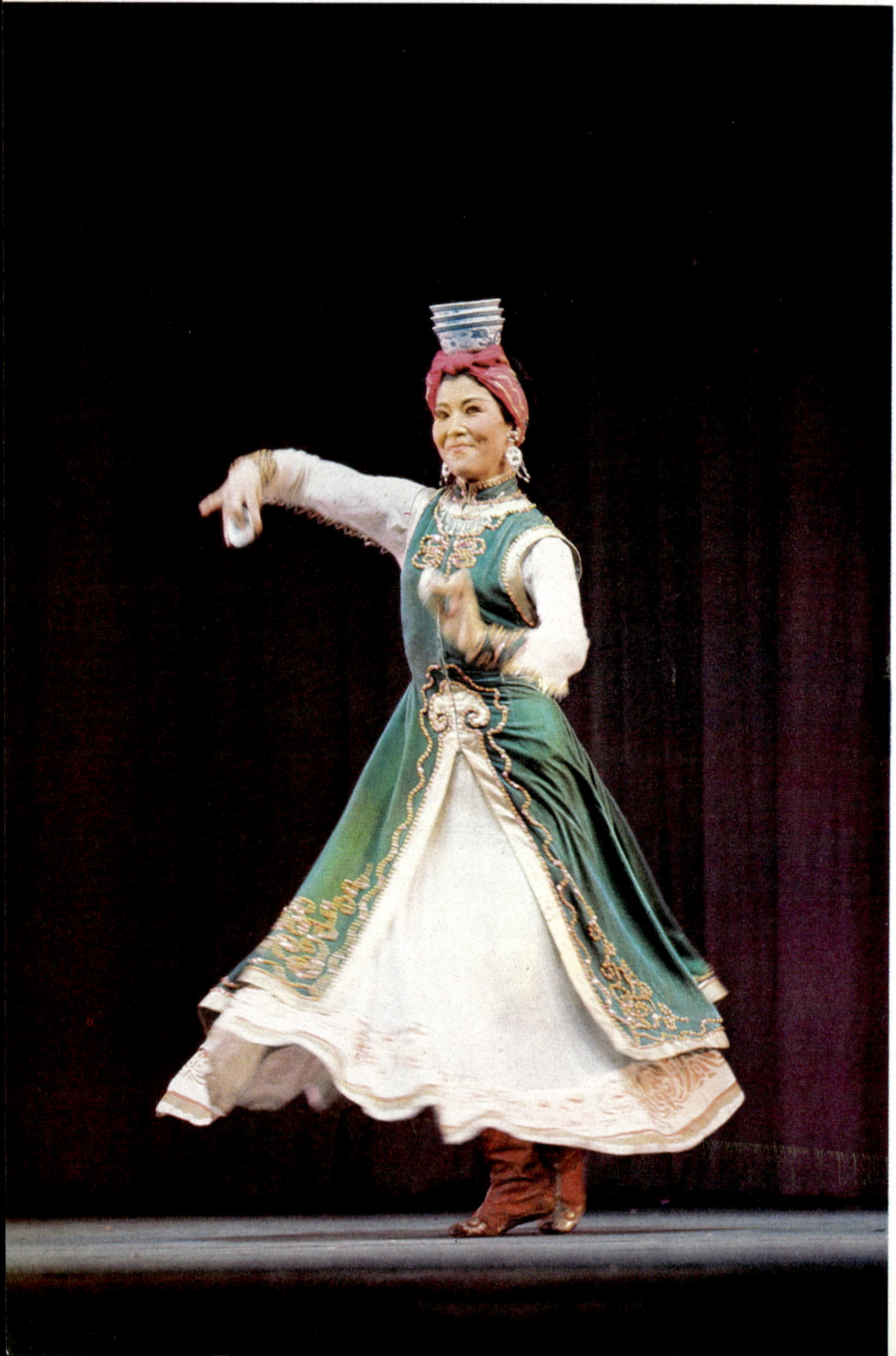

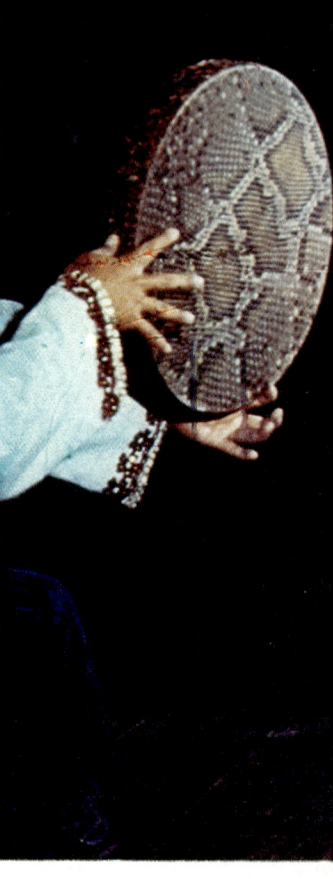

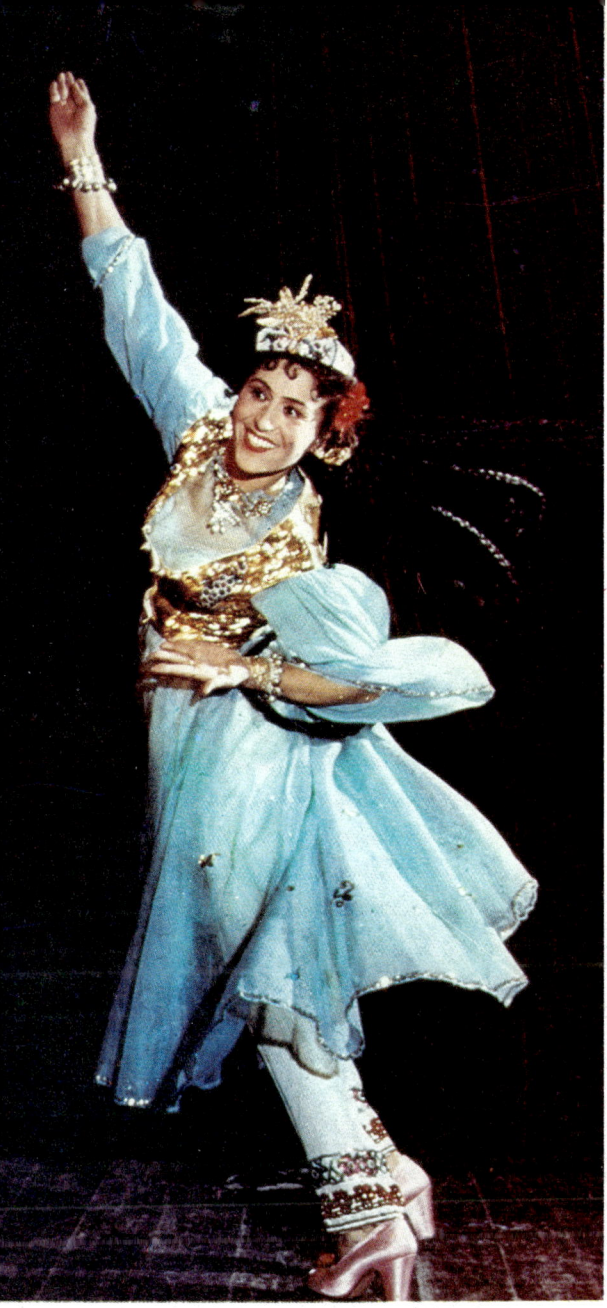

11. The Tatar dancer Zuohala performing the "Bell and Drum Dance".

10. The Uygur dancer Ayitula performing "Picking Grapes".

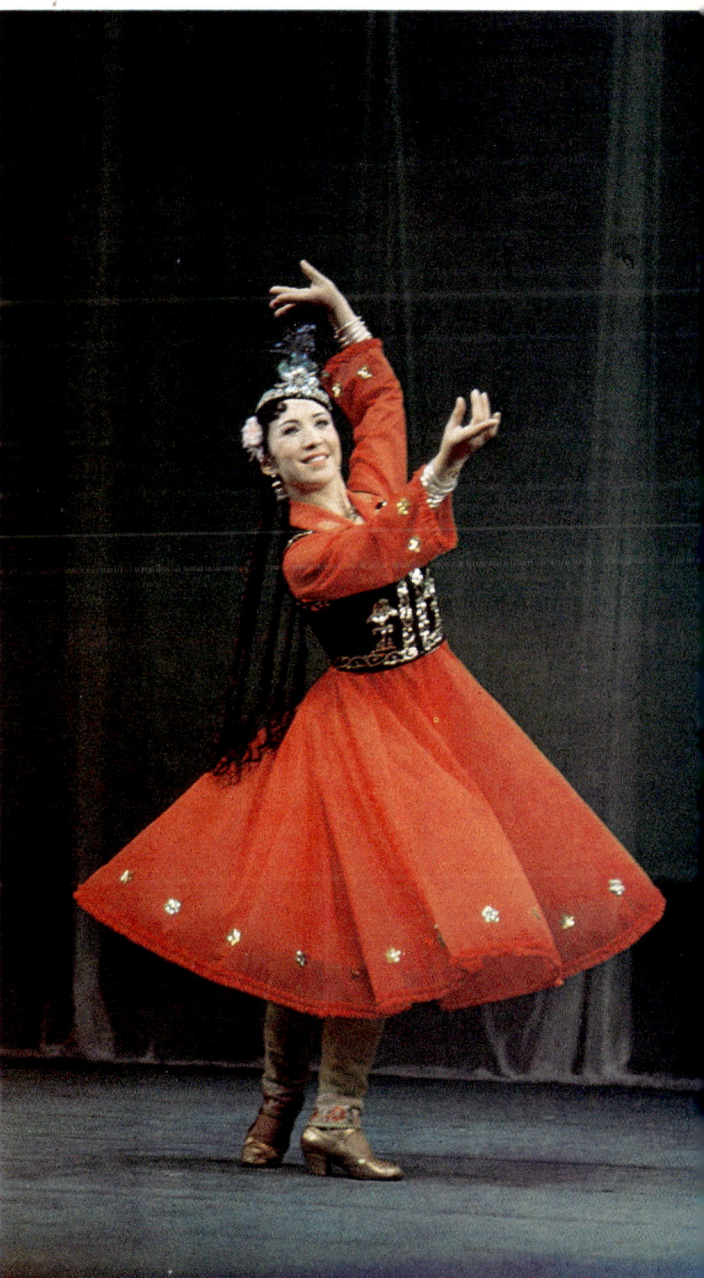

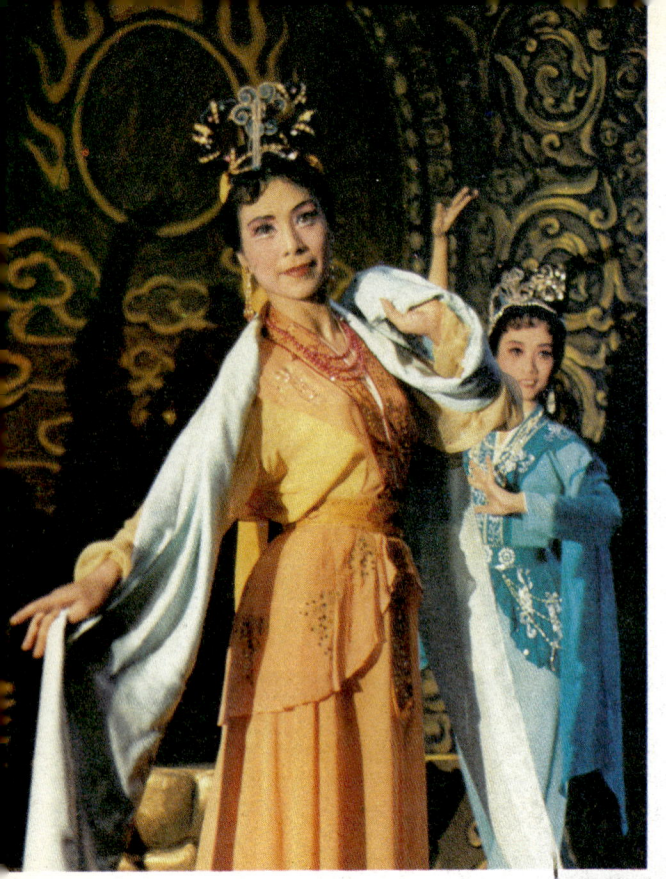

12. The Han dancer Zhao Qing playing Sanshengmu in the dance drama *Precious Lotus Lamp*.

13. The "Long Silk Dance" from the dance drama *Precious Lotus Lamp*.

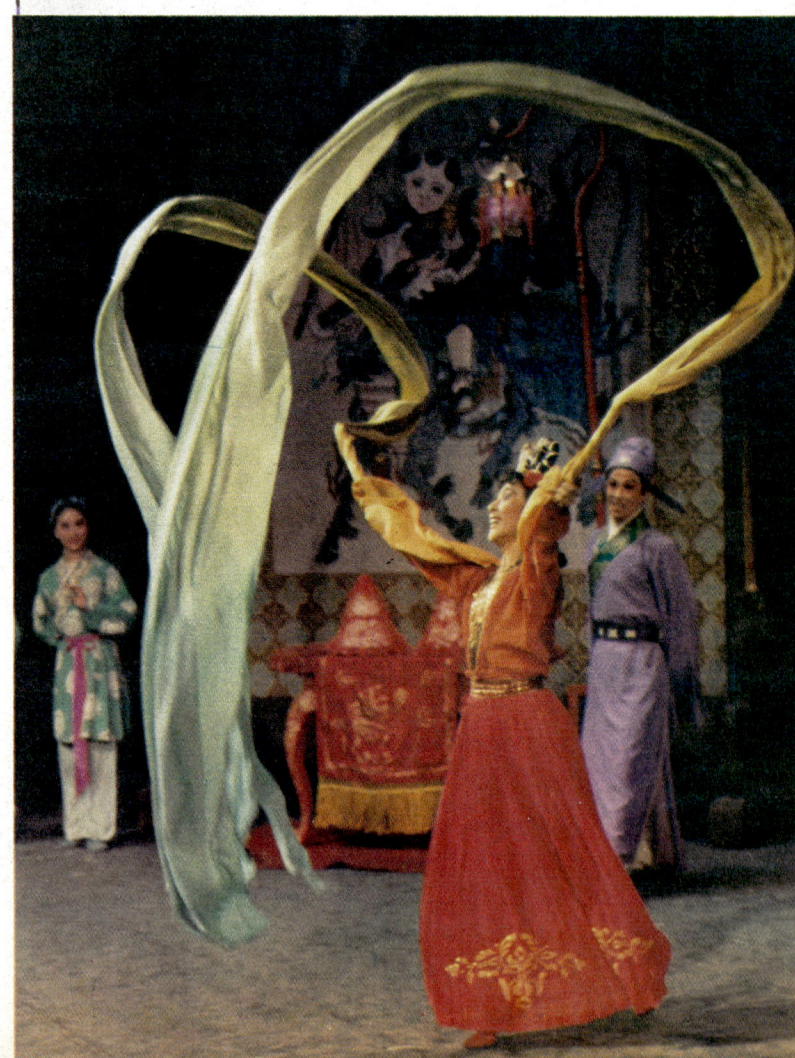

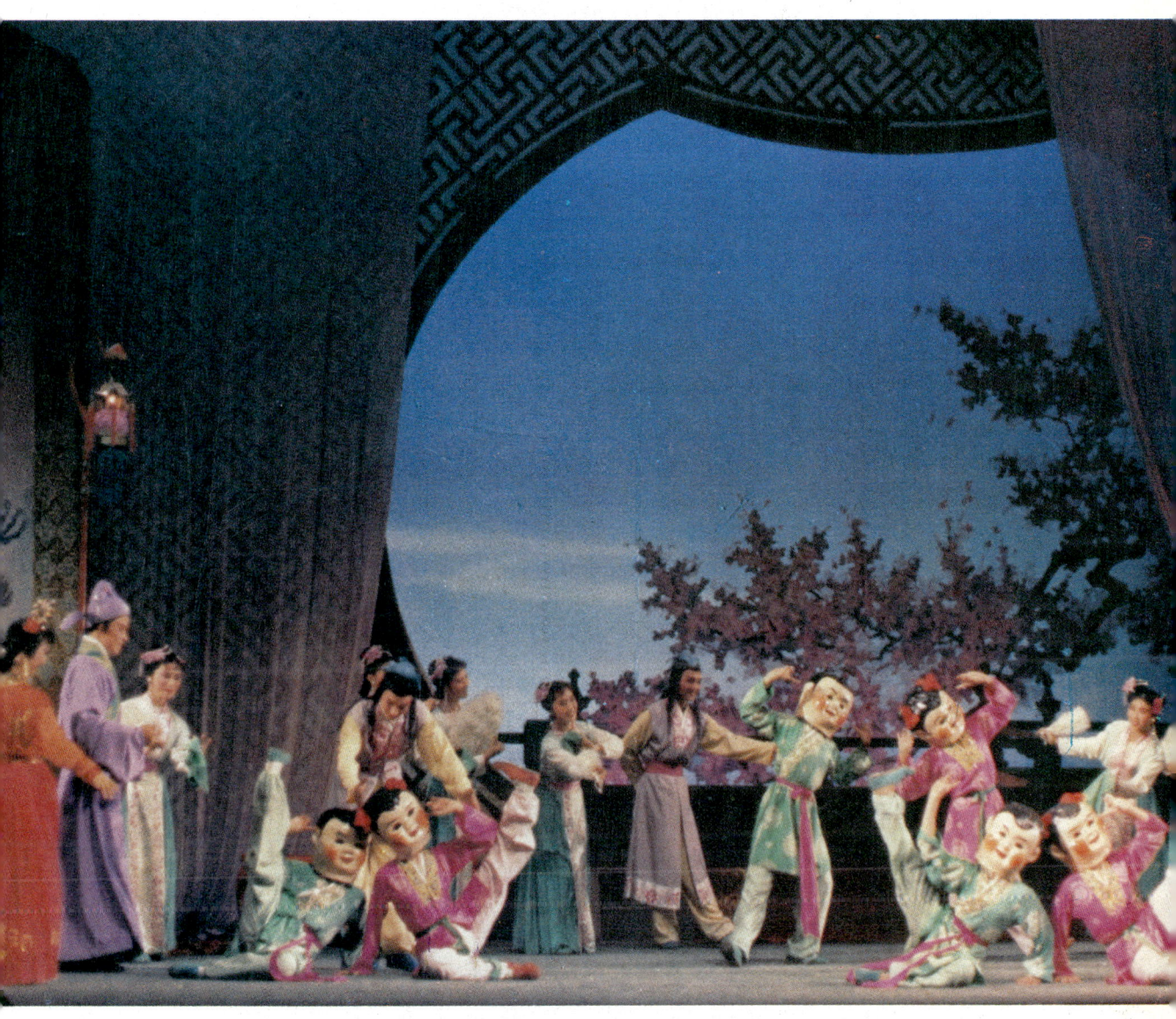

14. The "Big Head Dance" from the dance drama *Precious Lotus Lamp*.

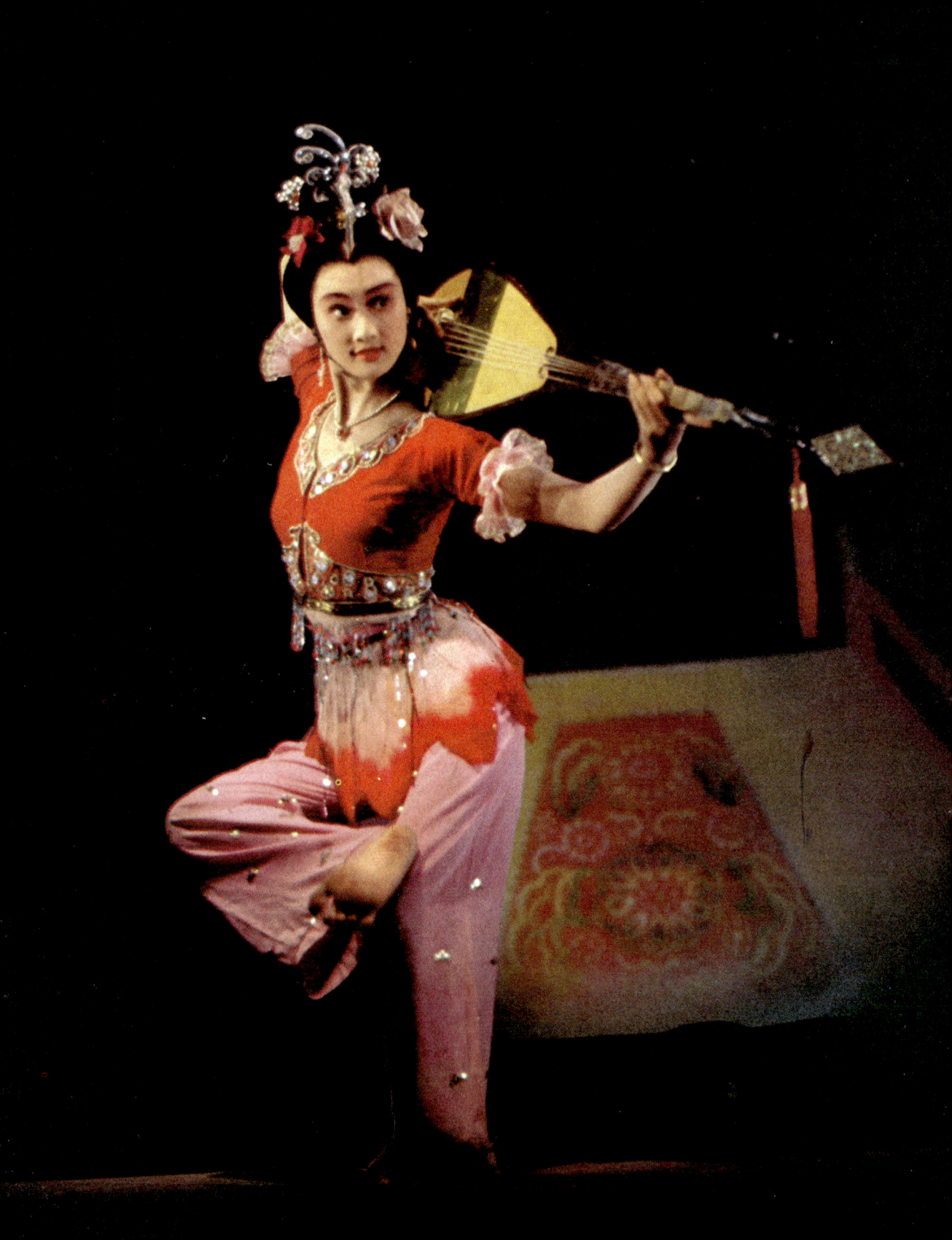

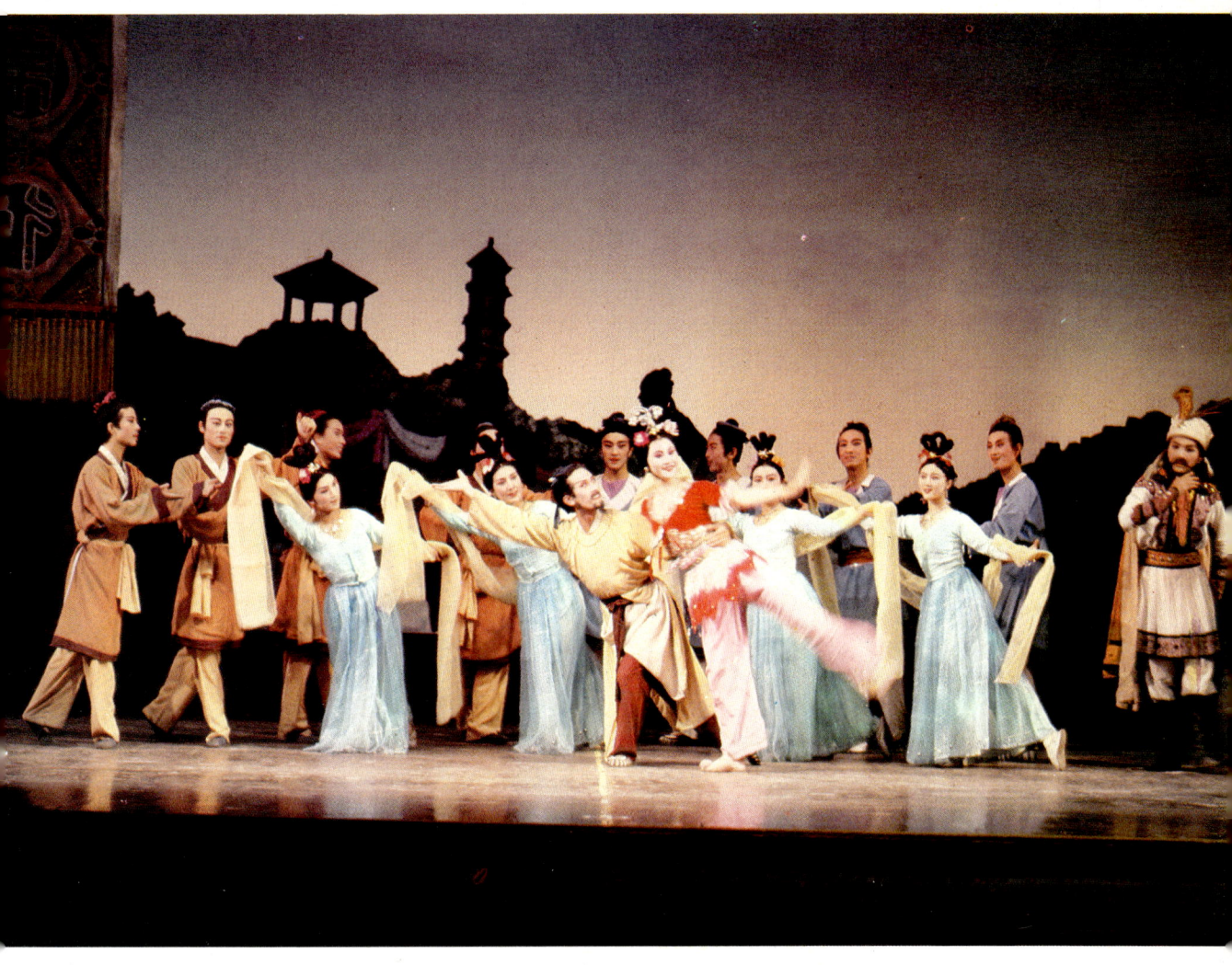

16. A scene from the dance drama *Rain of Flowers on the Silk Road*.

15. Yingniang, the heroine in the dance drama *Rain of Flowers on the Silk Road* performing "Playing the *Pipa* Backwards".

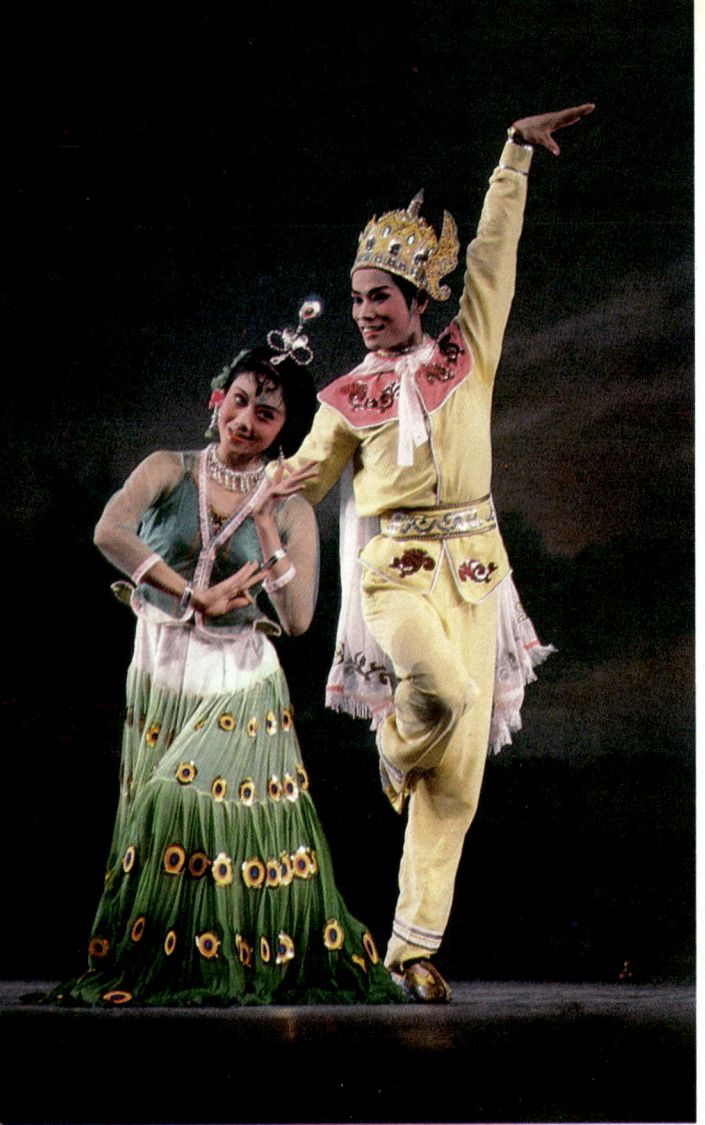

17. A pas de deux by the male and female leads in the dance drama *Zhaoshutun and Nanmuruona*.

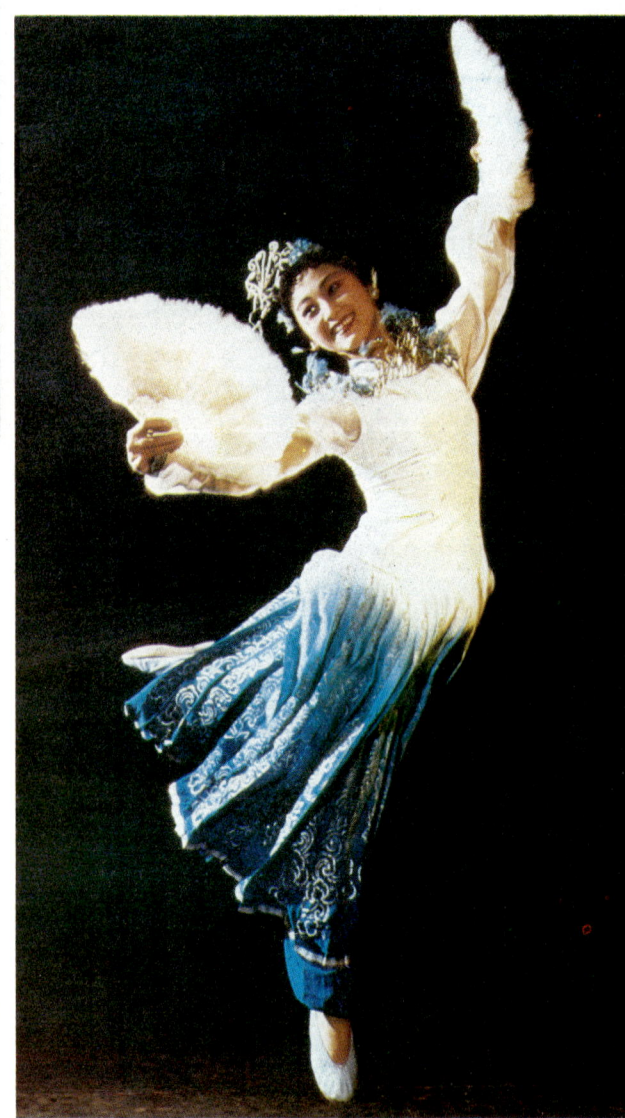

18. The Han dancer Chen Ailian performing "A Moonlit Spring Night by the River of Flowers".

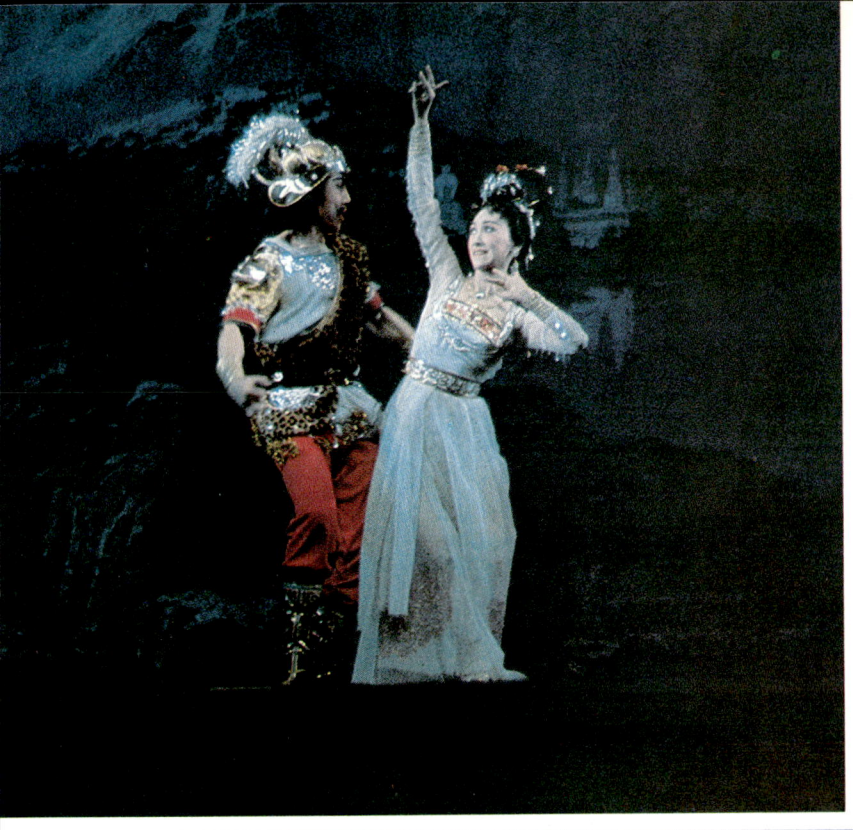

19. Chen Ailian playing the title role in the dance drama *Princess Wencheng*.

20. A scene from the dance drama *Princess Wencheng*.

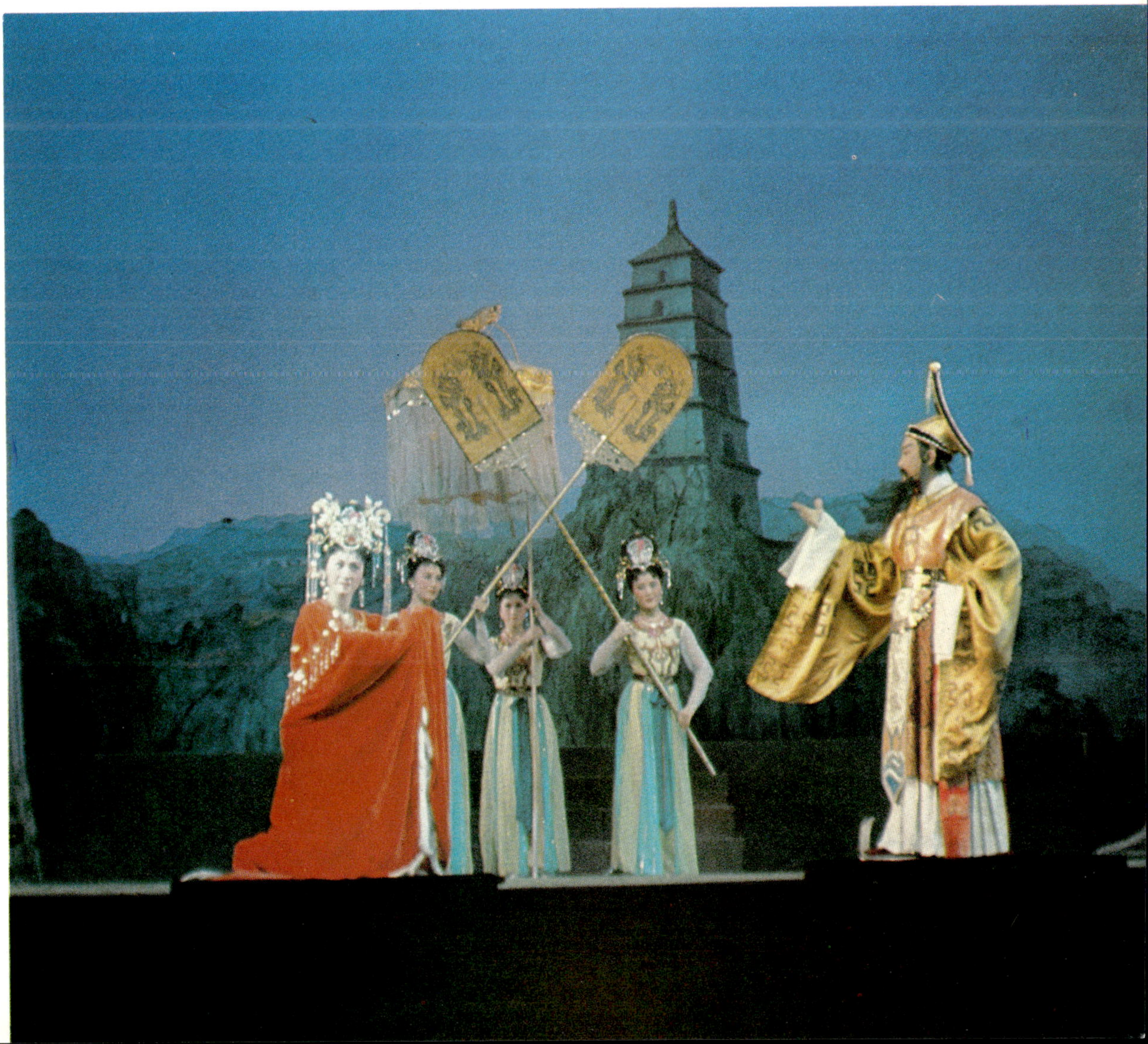

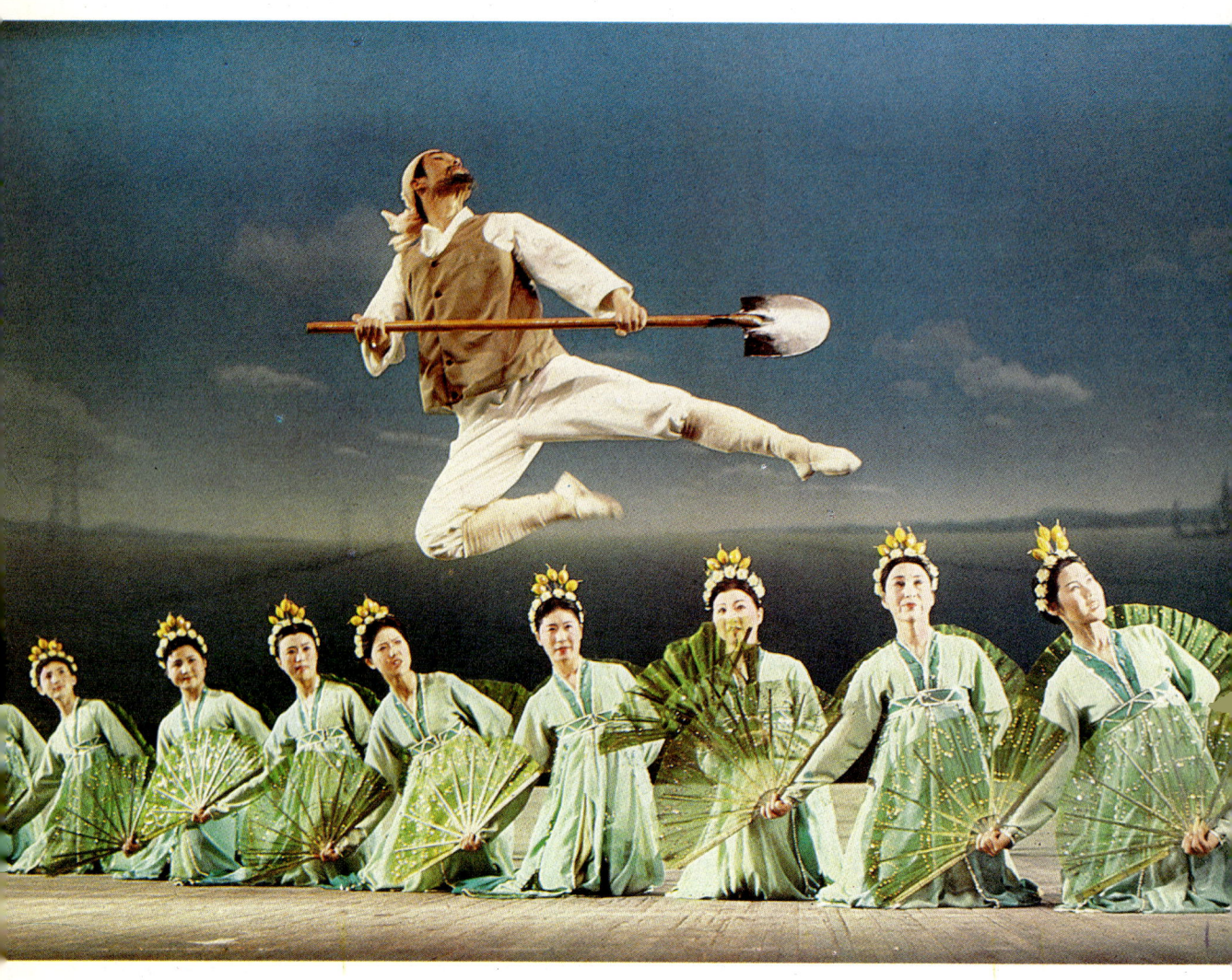
21. "The Waterkeepers"   (Korean).

22. "Battle Drum of Golden Mountain" (Han).

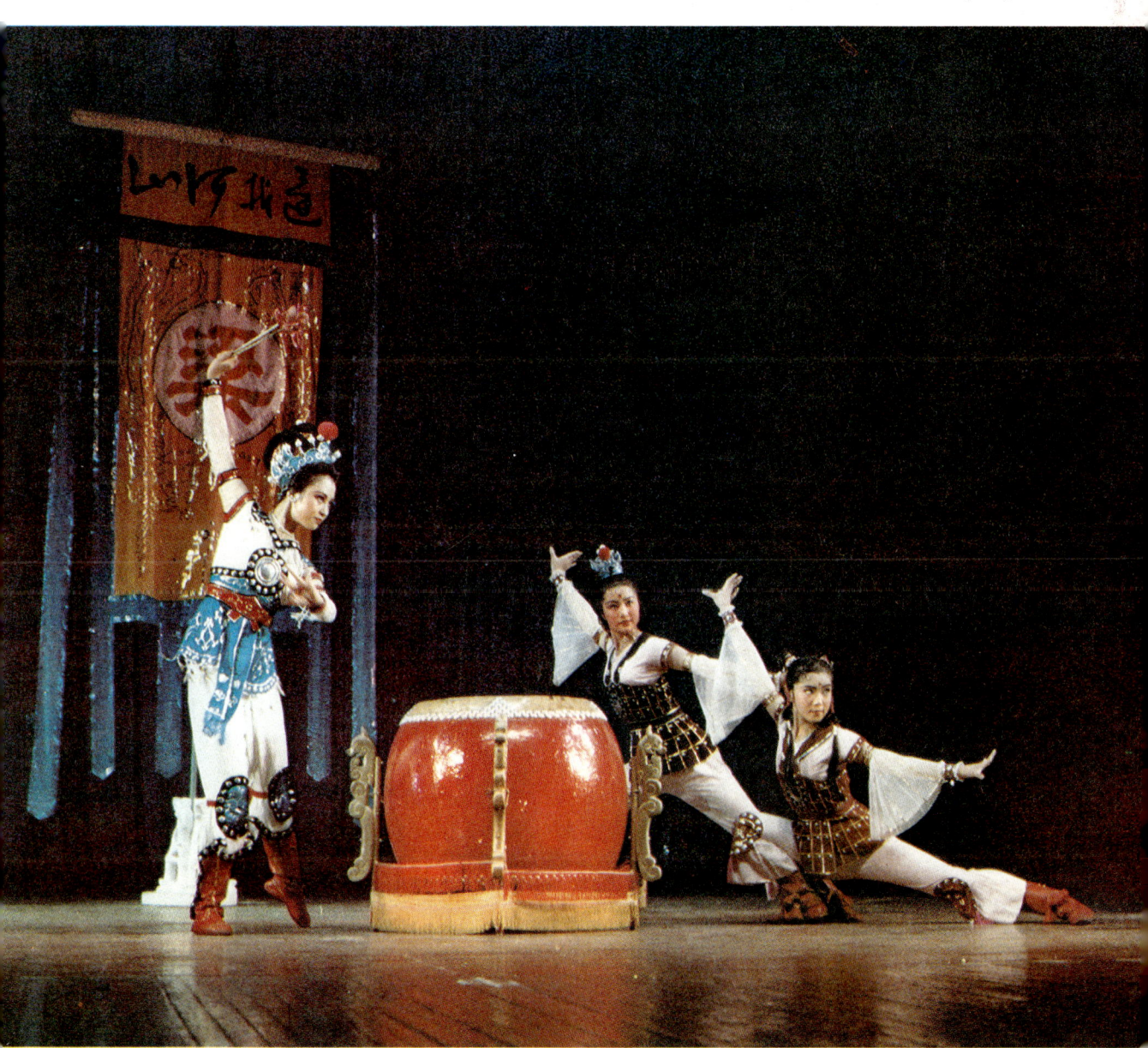

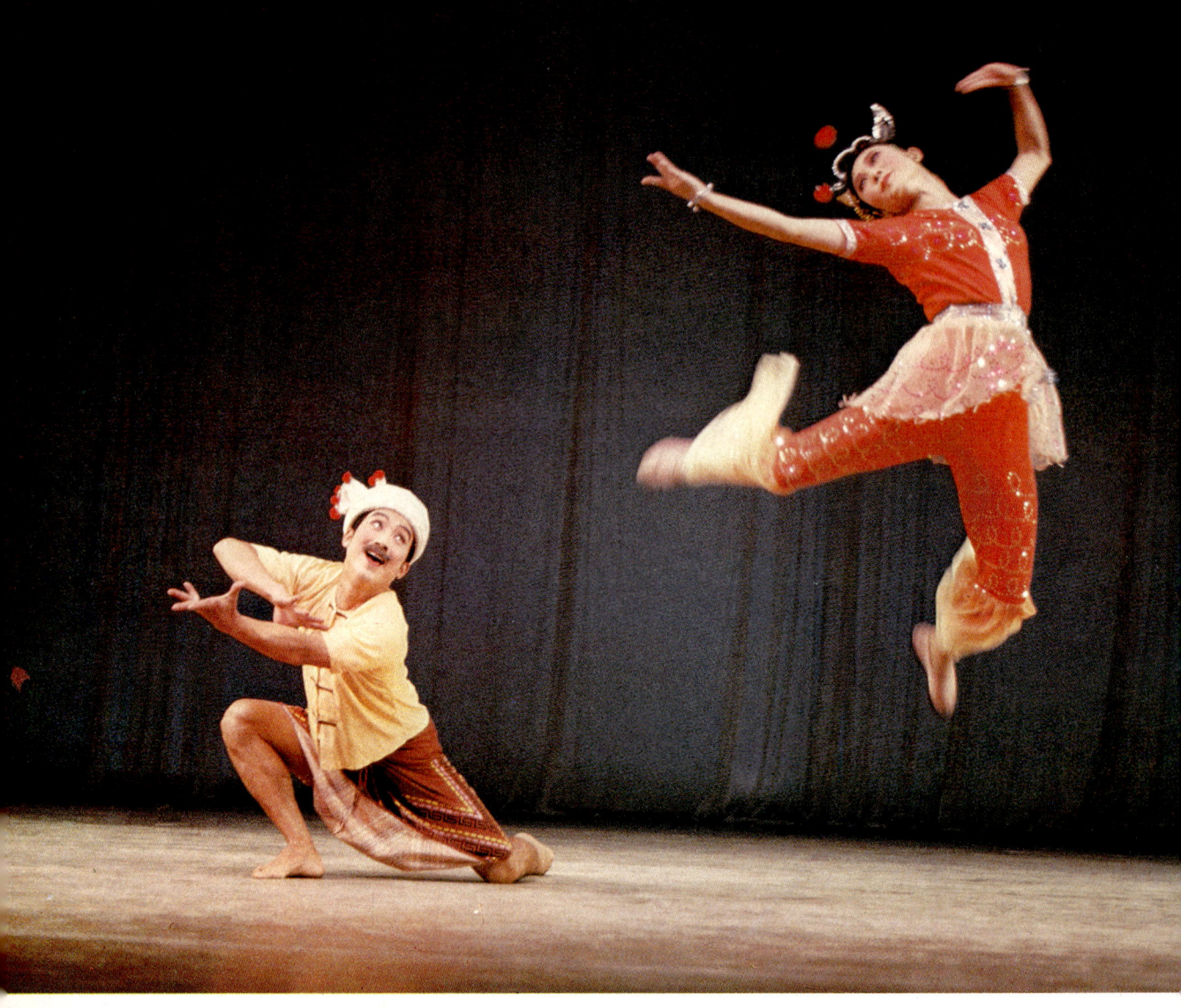

23. "Catching Fish" (Dai).

24. The Dai dancer Dao Meilan performing "Water".

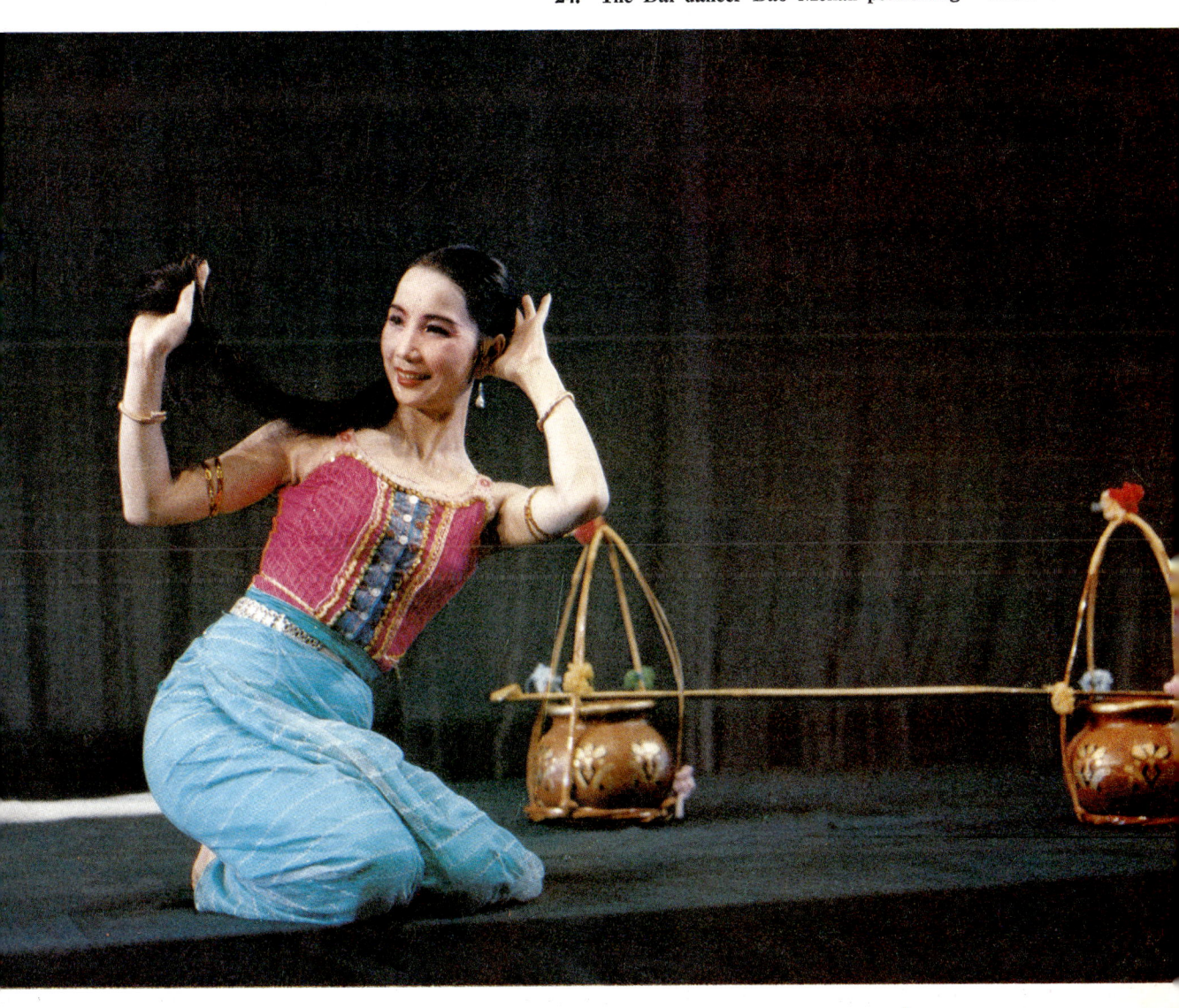

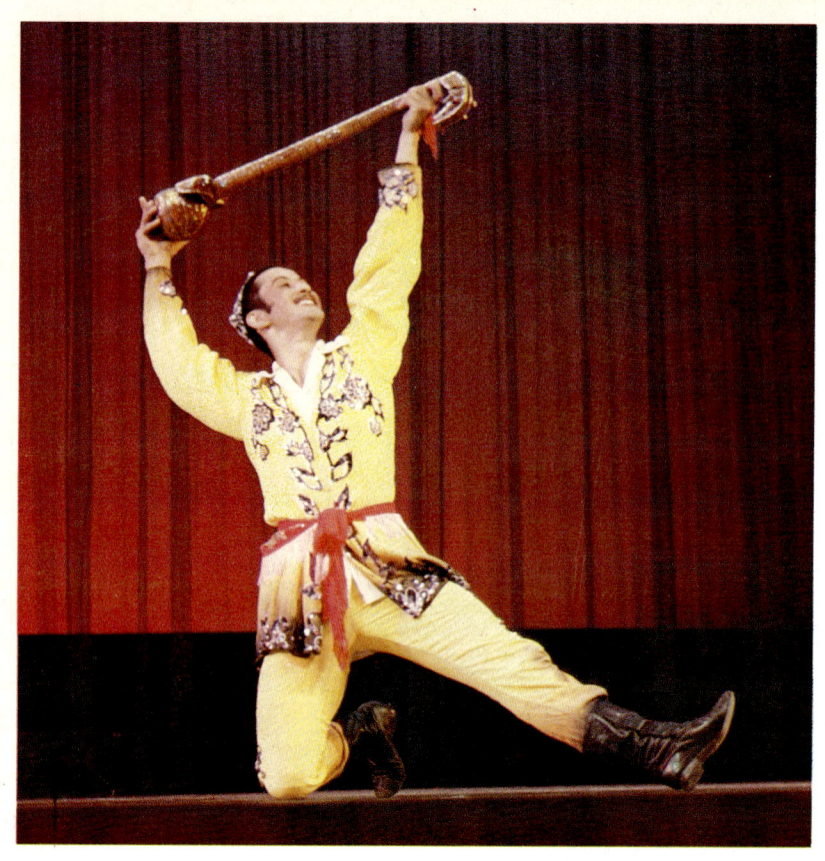

25. "My Rewafu"   (Uygur).

26. "Happy Linka"   (Tibetan).

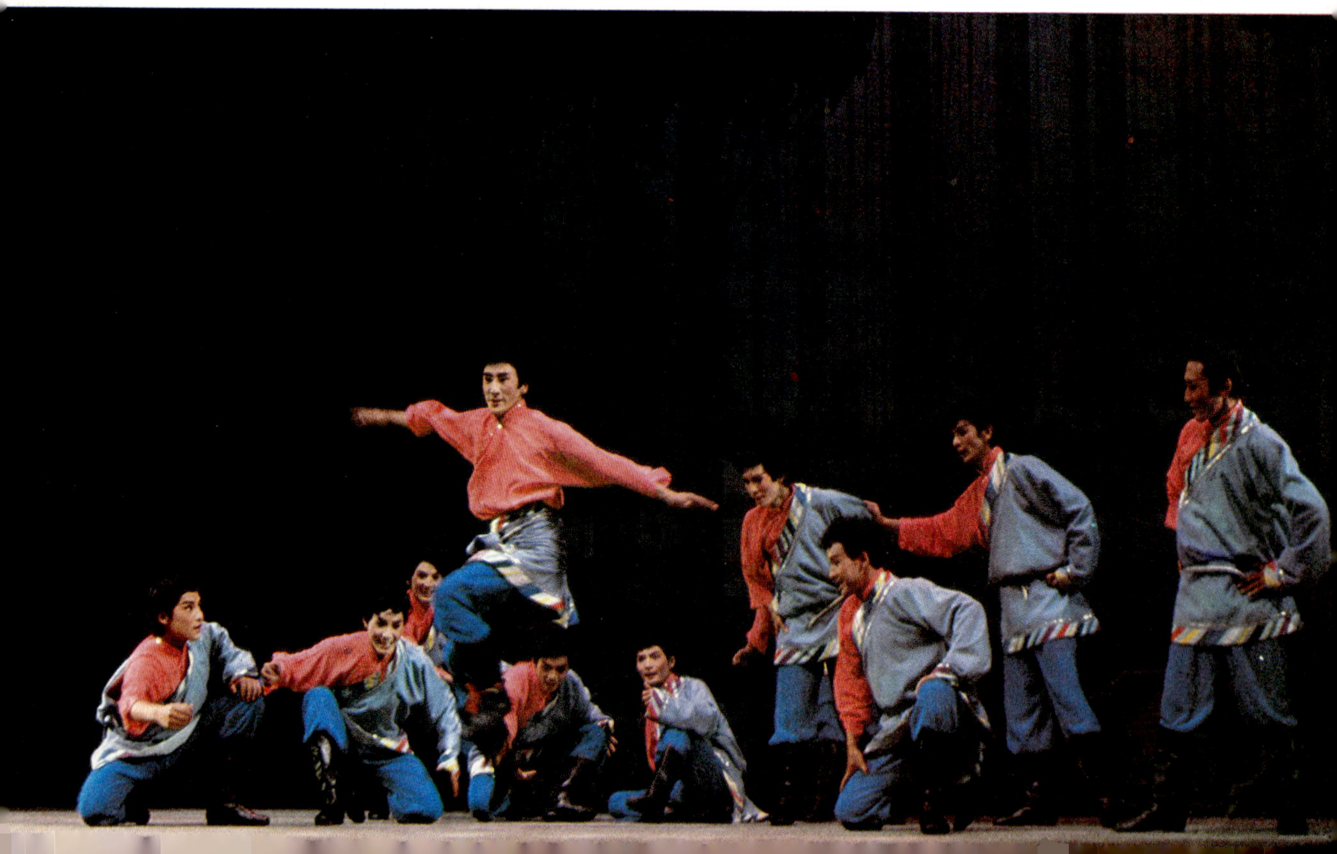

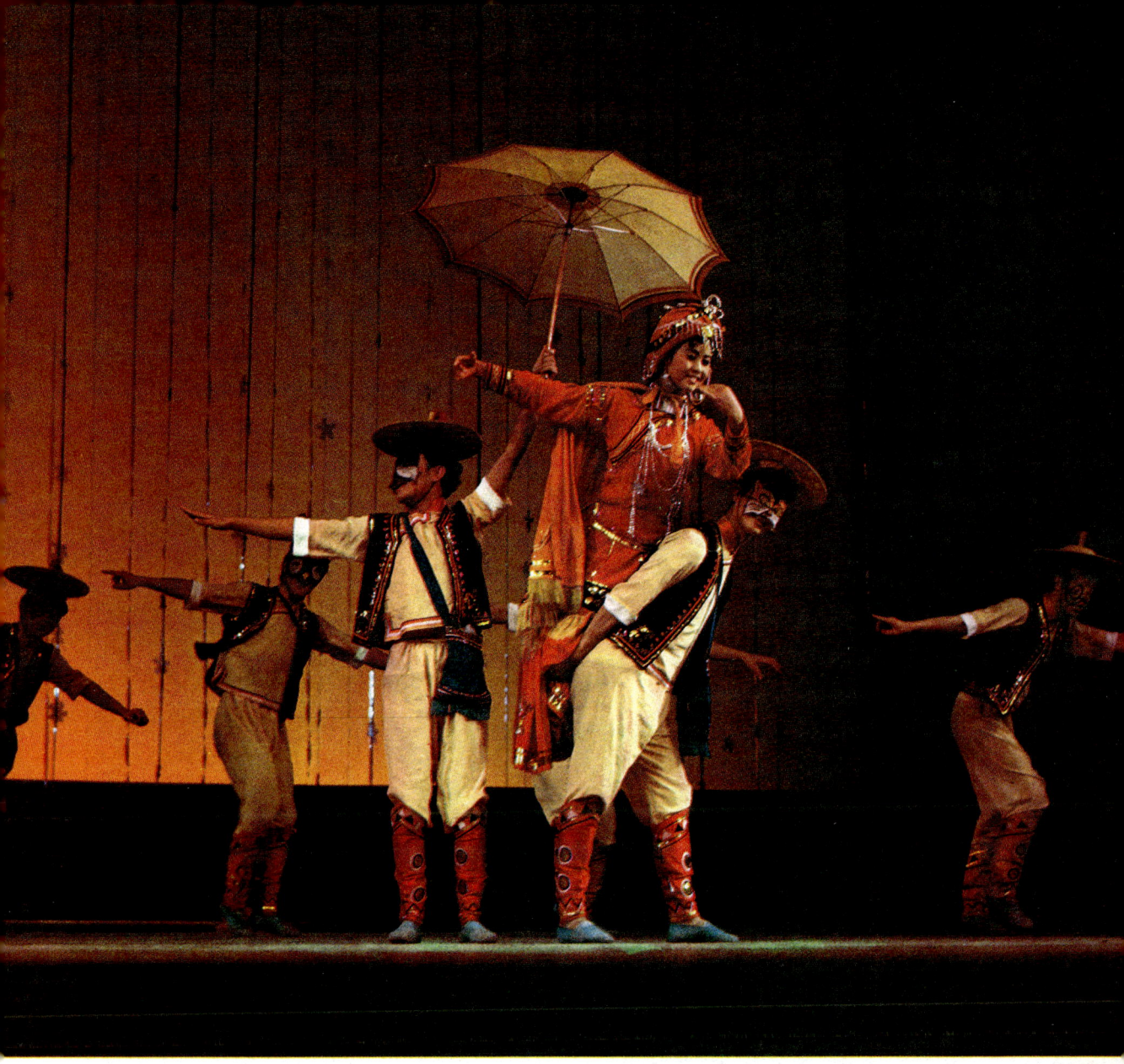

27. "A Piggyback for the Bride"　(Yi).

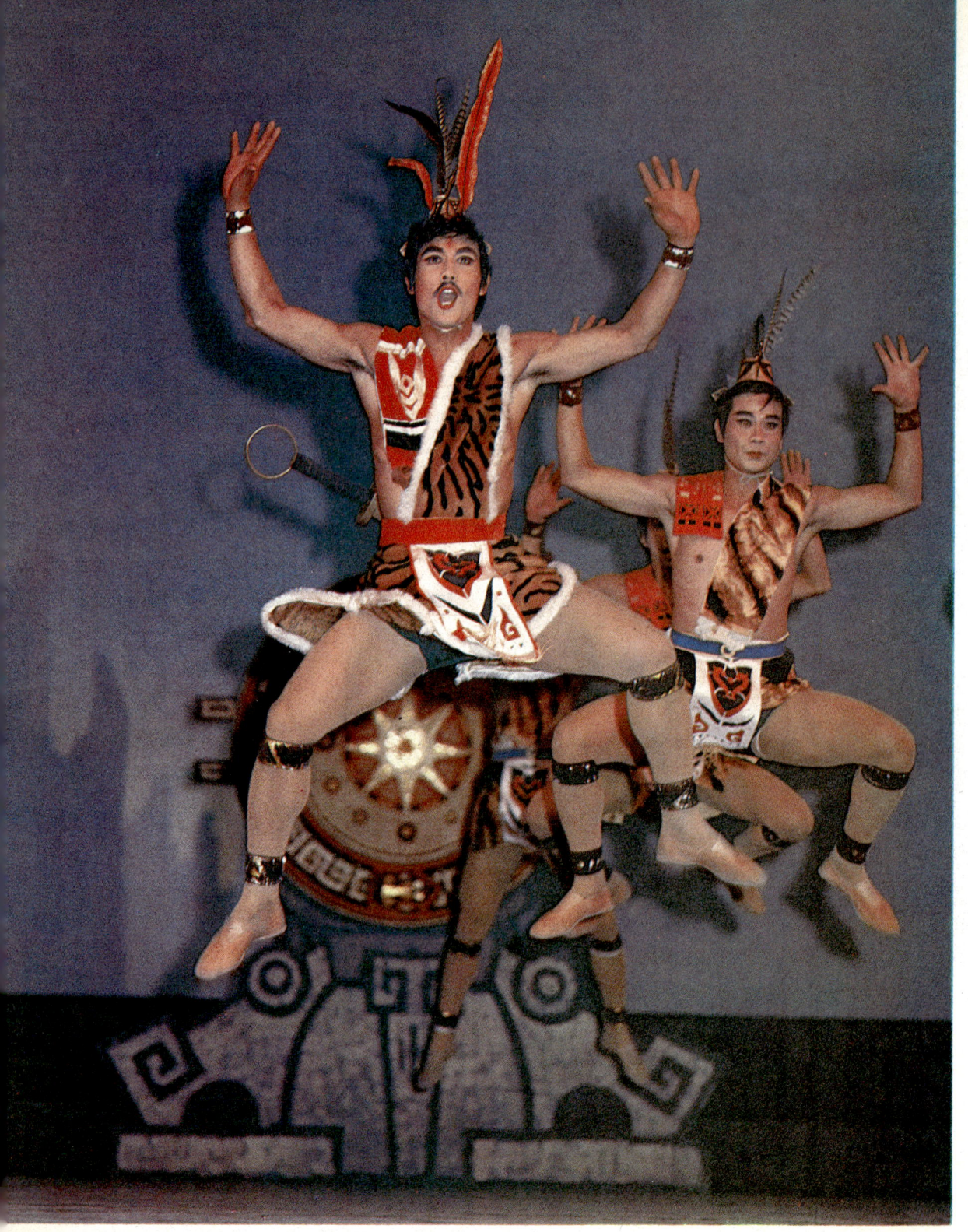

28. "Battle Drum of Huashan" (Zhuang).

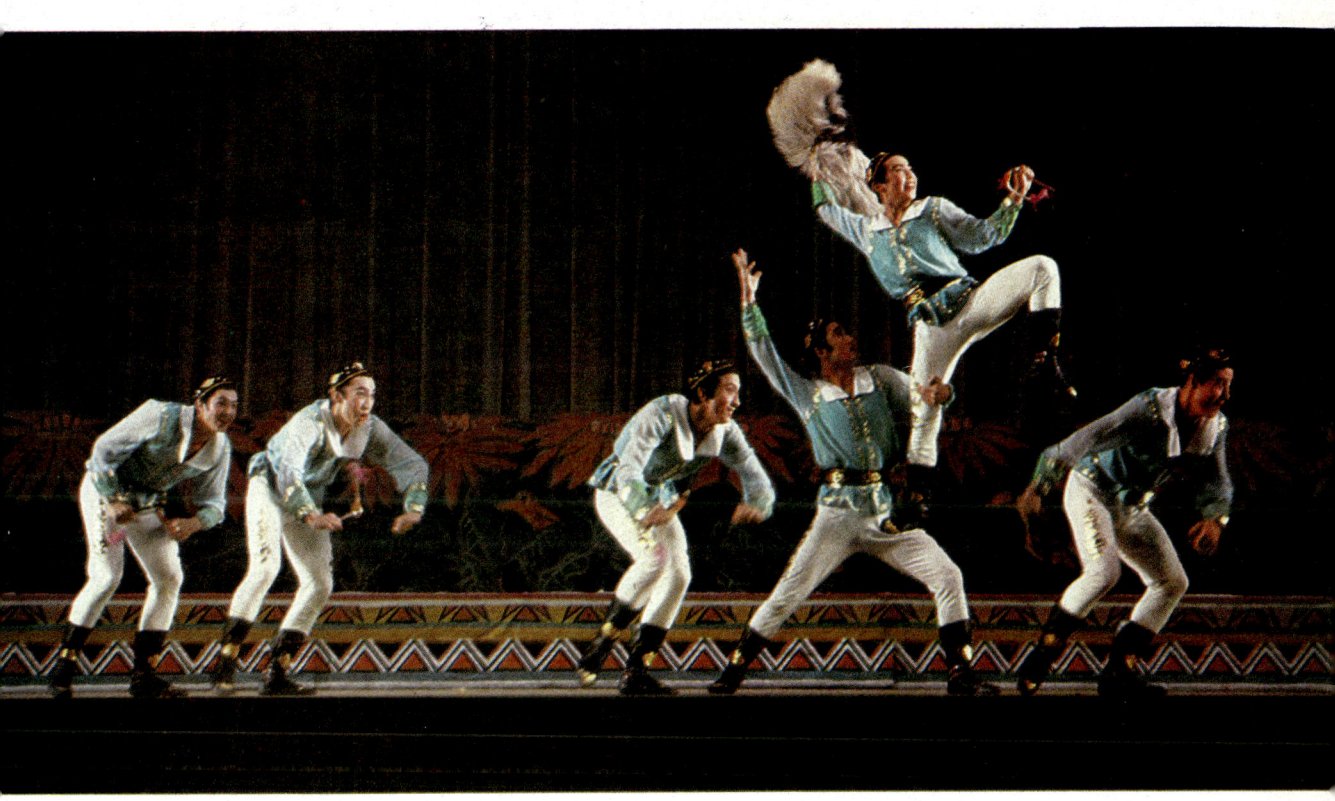

29. "Goat-Picking Dance" (Kazak).

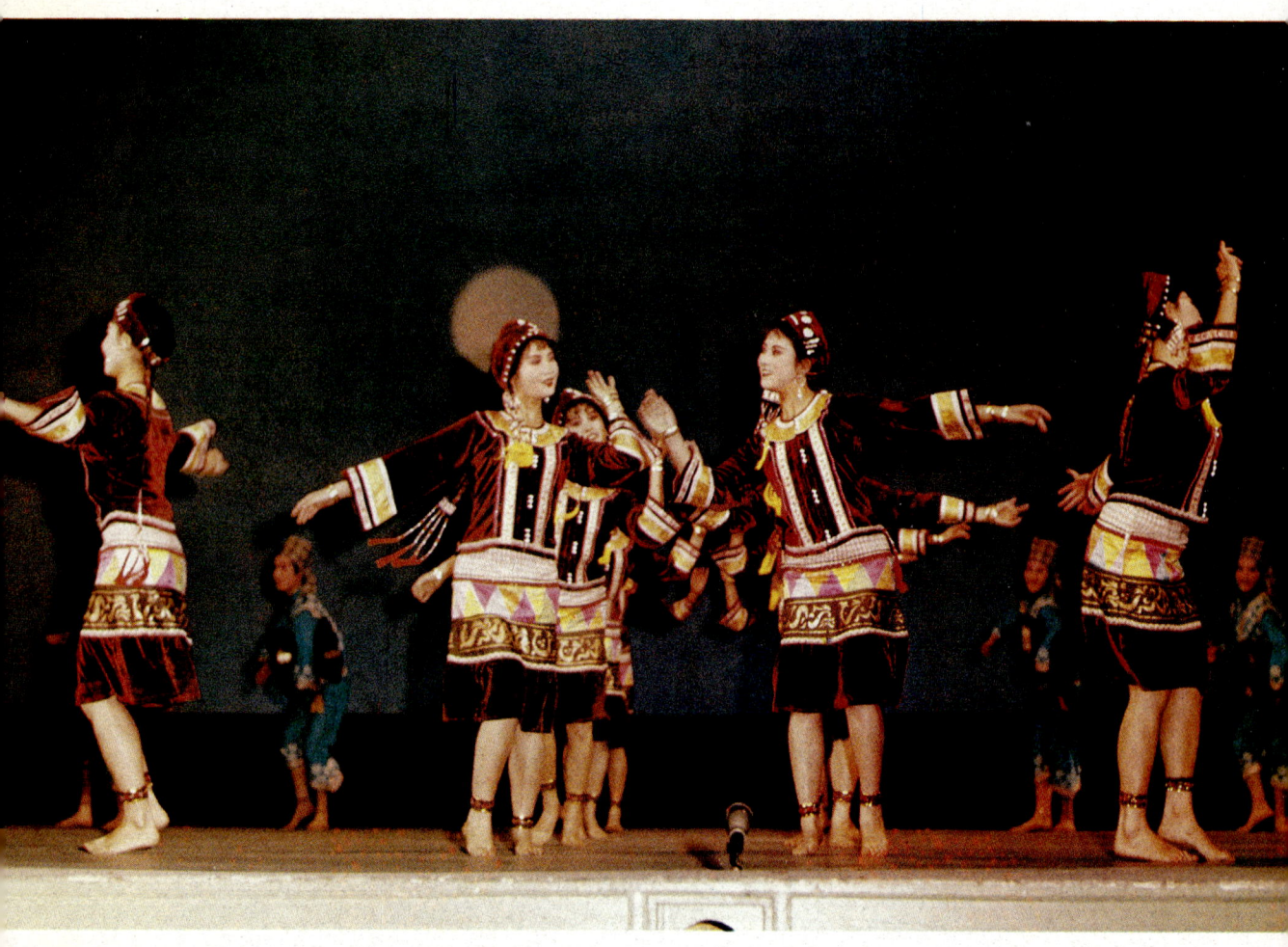

30. "Bronze Drum Dance"   (Yi).

31. "Tending the Lion" (Tibetan).

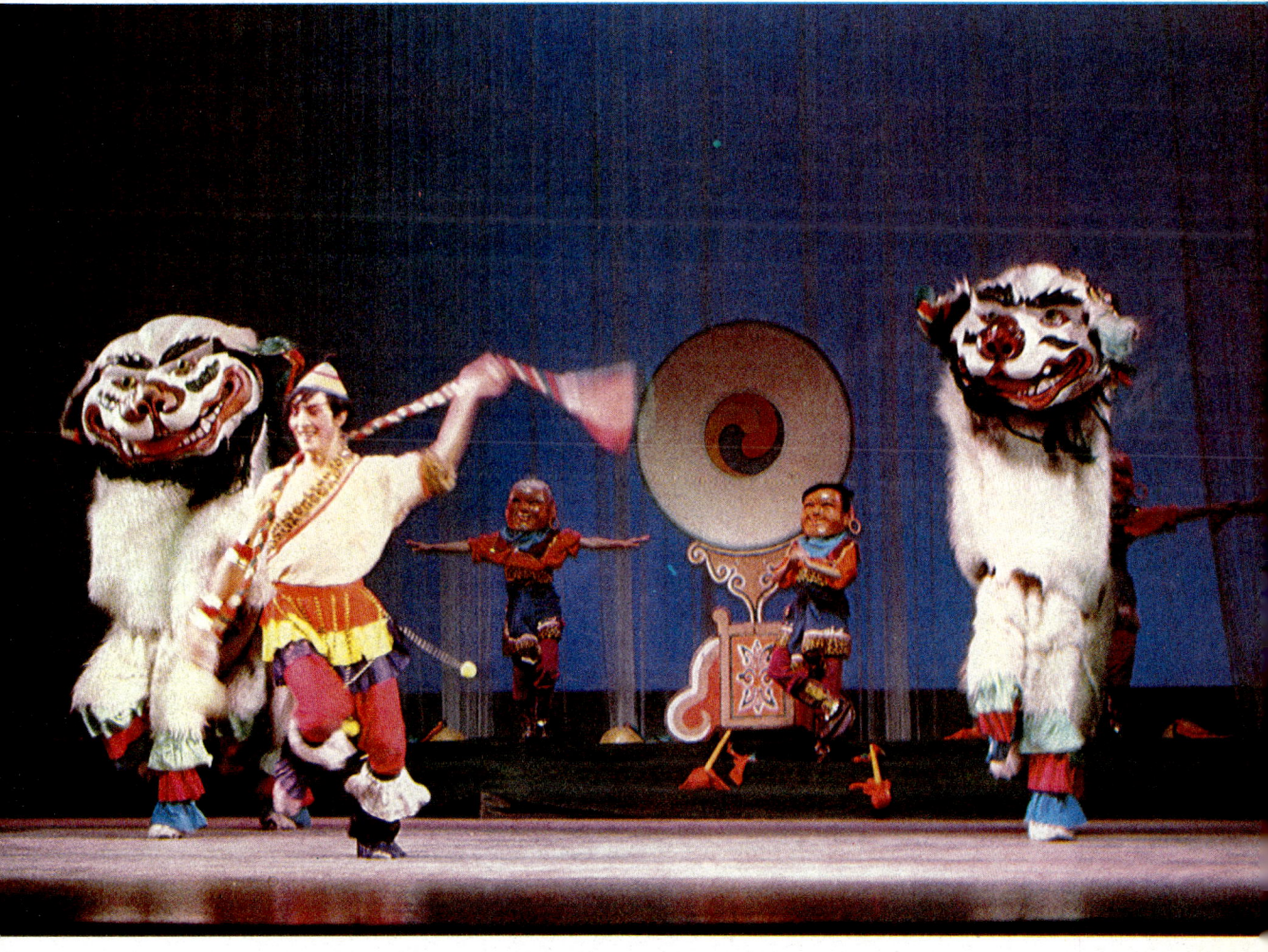

32. "Springtime for Xiaerba" (Xiaerba from the region of Tibet).

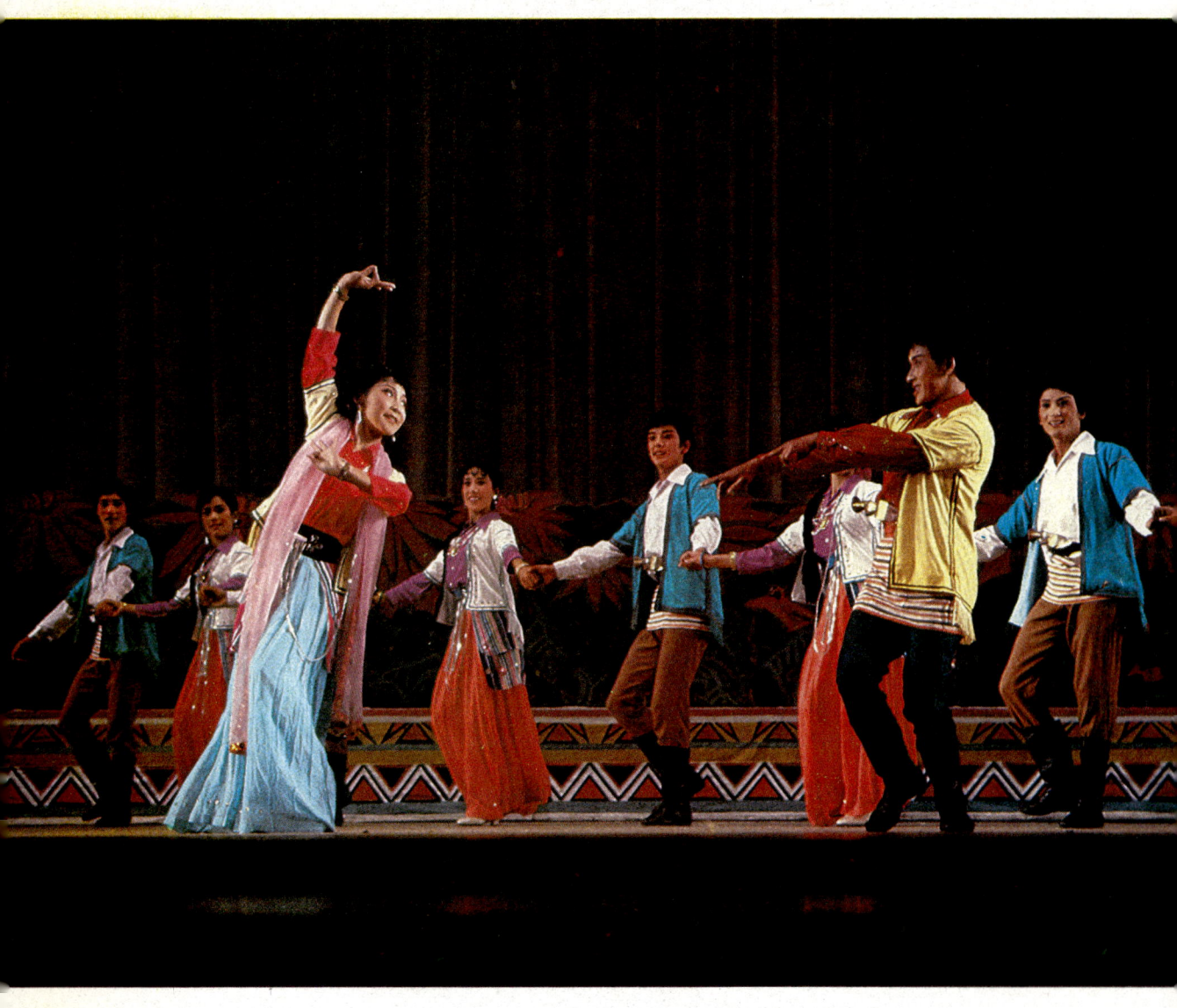

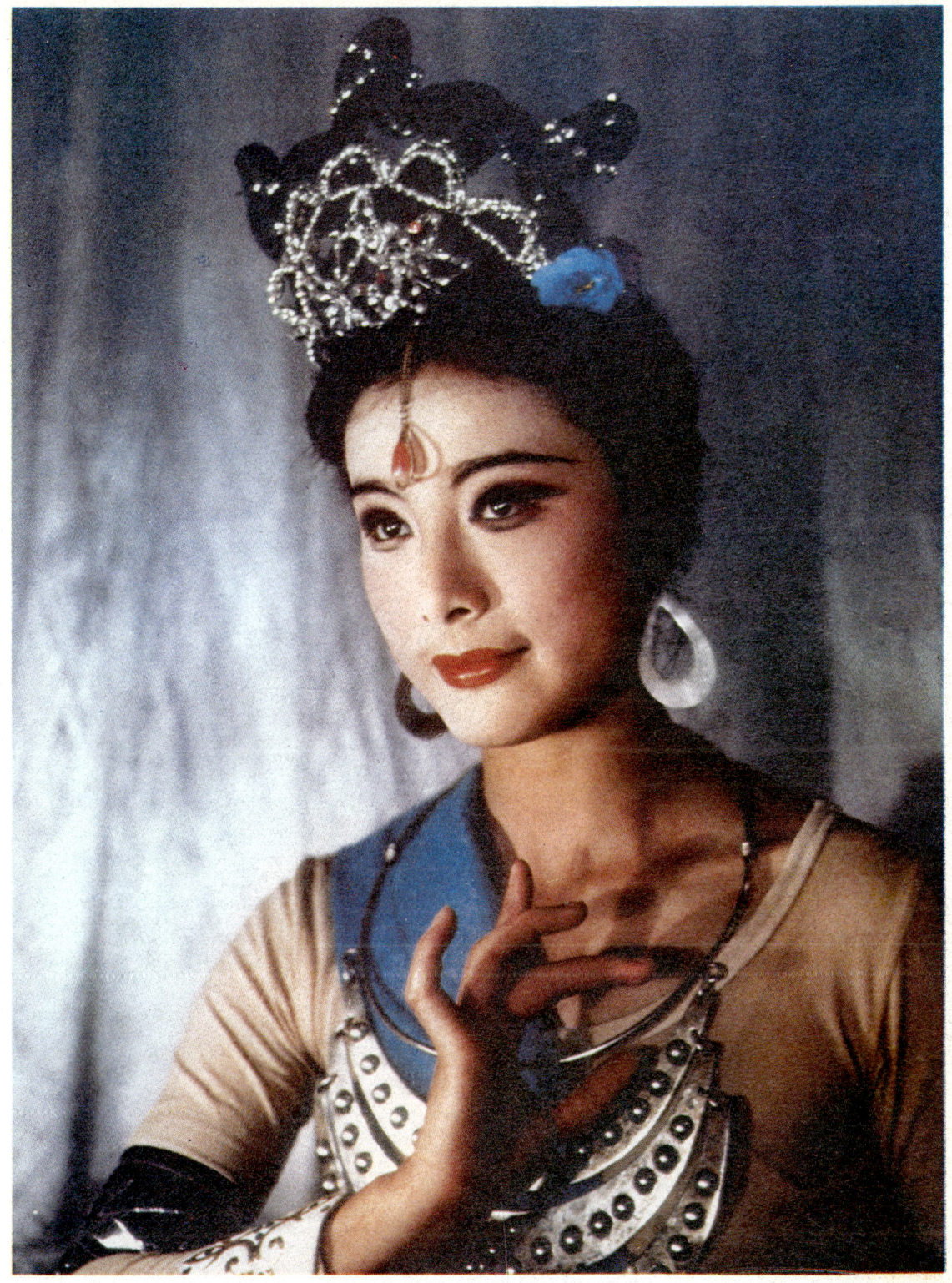

33. "Painted Sculptures from Dunhuang" (Han).

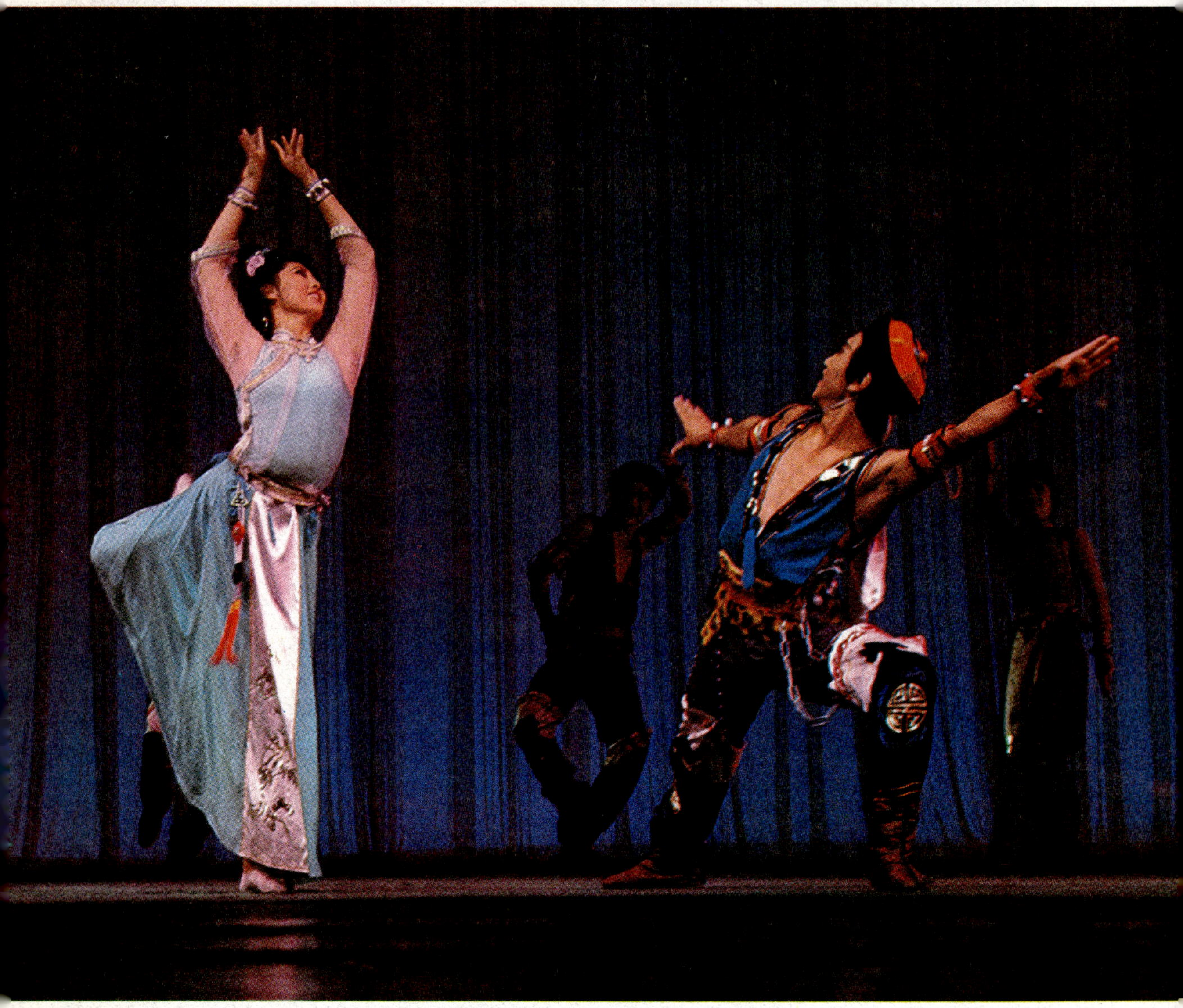

34. "Mangshi Kongqi"   (Manchu).

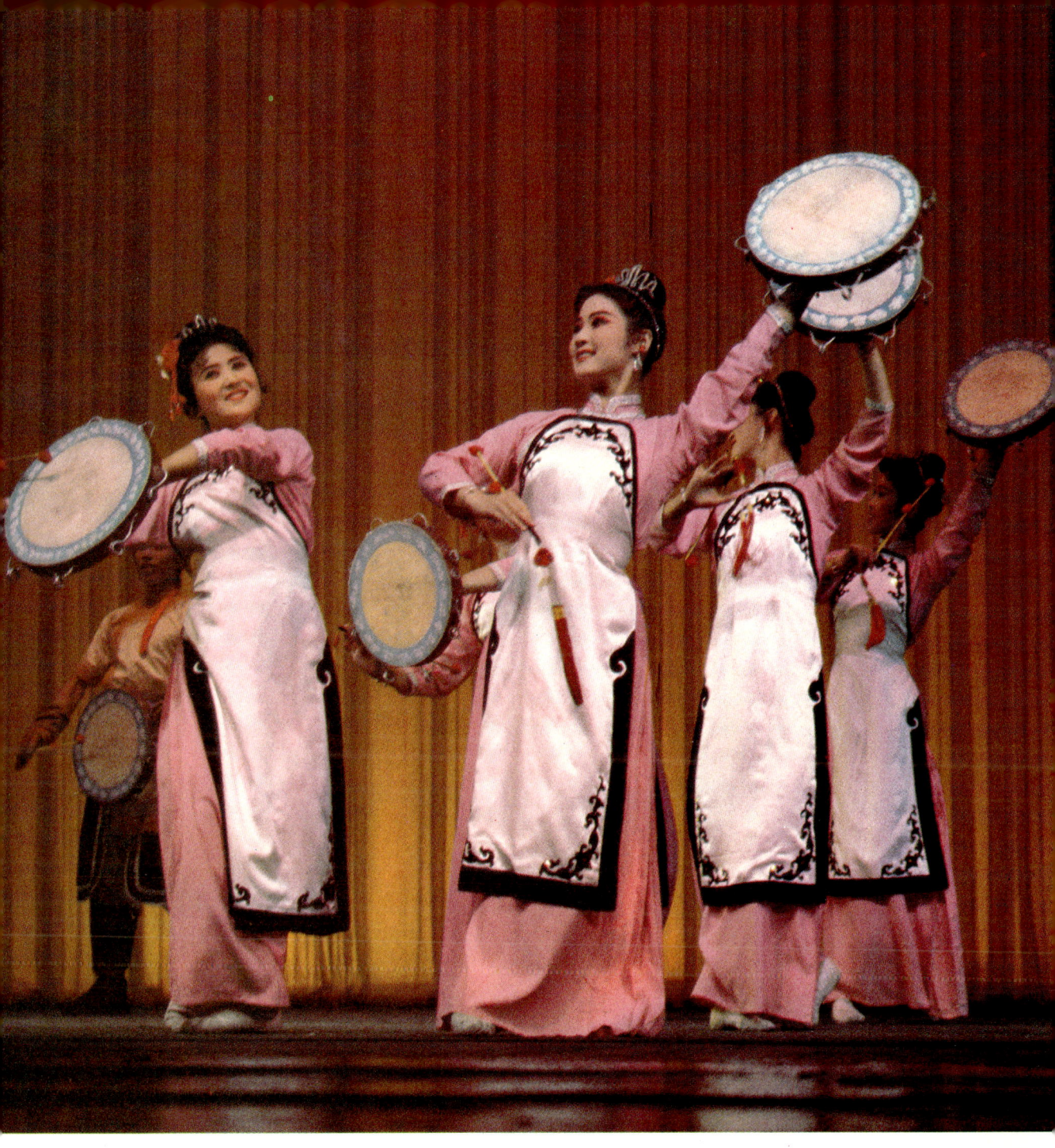

35. "Drum Dance"　(Manchu).

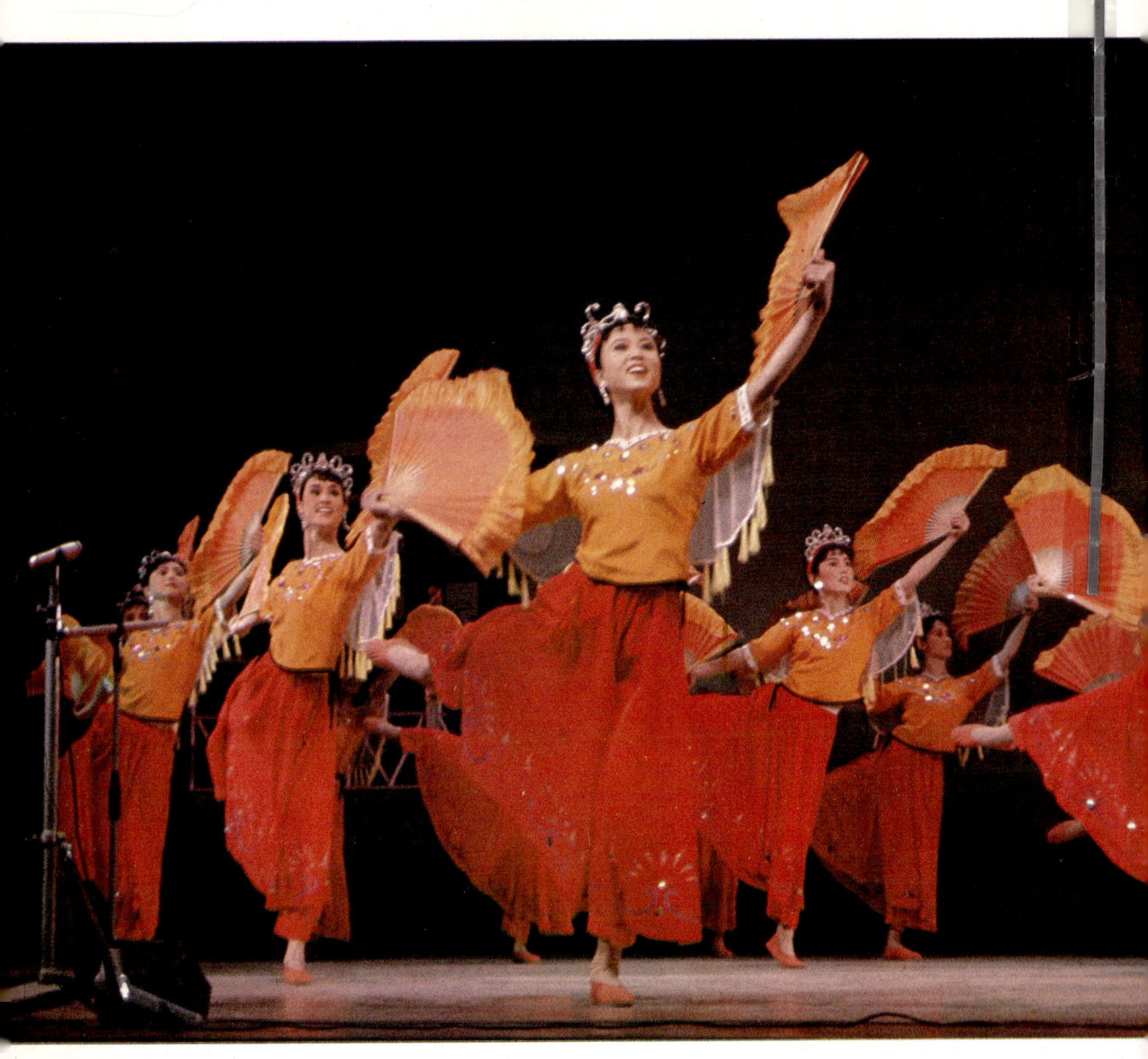

36. "The Furnace Burns Brighter" (Miao).

37. "Muddy Legs" (Miao).

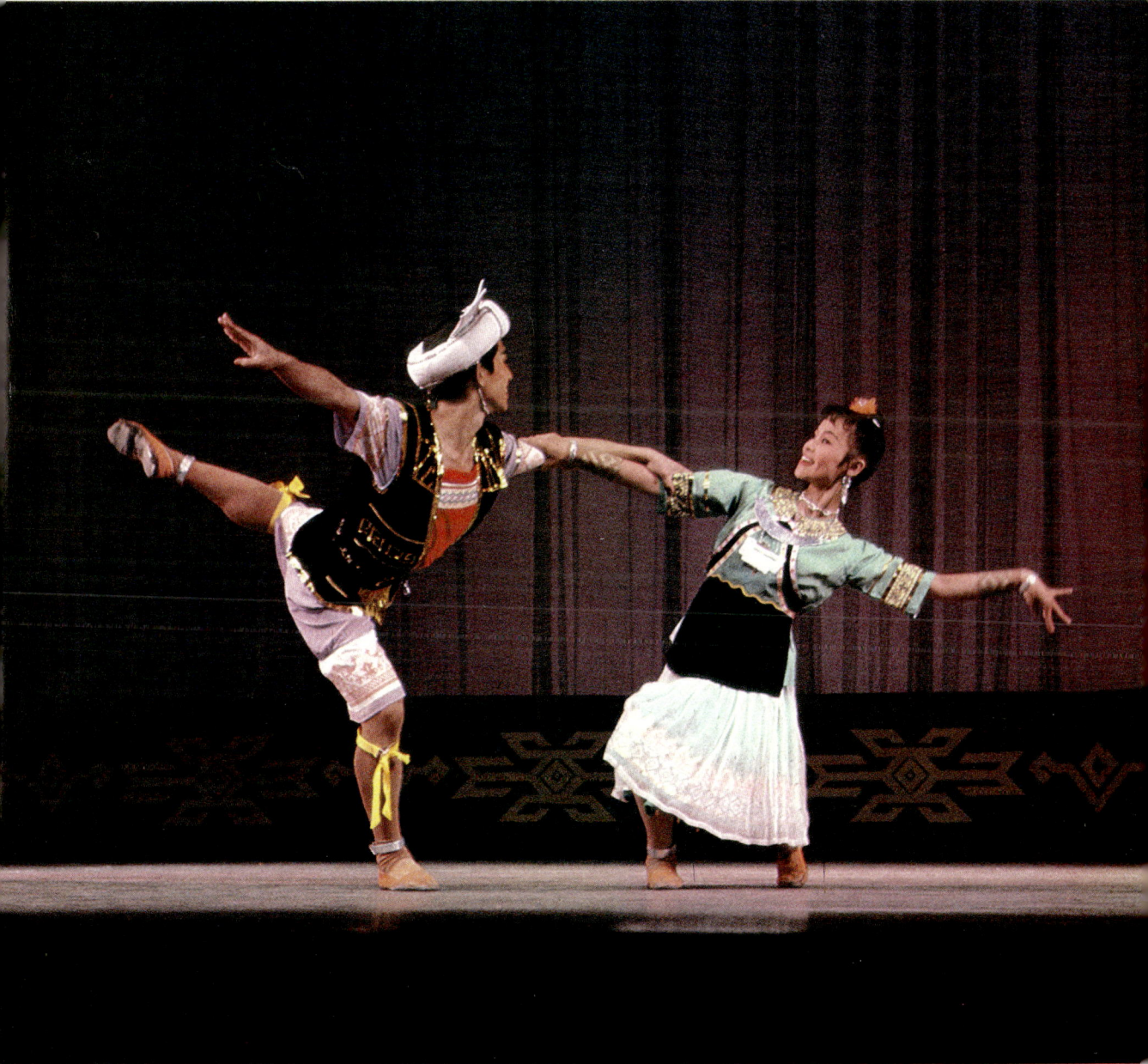

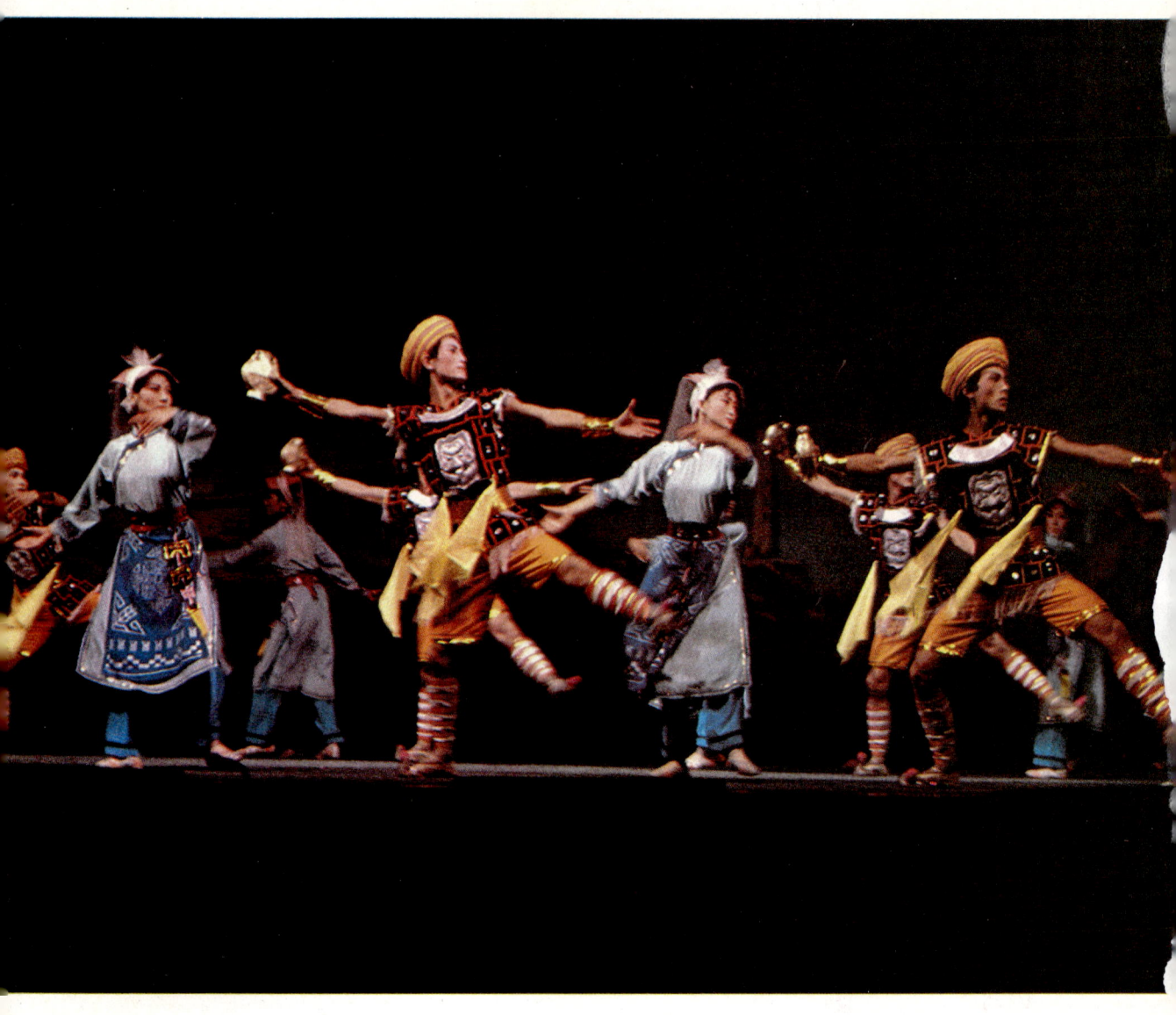

38. "Armour Dance" (Qiang).